Rethinking the Electronic Healthcare Record

Why the Electronic Healthcare Record failed so hard, and how it should be redesigned to support doctors and nurses effectively in their work.

Dr. J. Martin Wehlou, MD, CISSP

MITM Books

MAN IN THE MIDDLE BOOKS

First published in book form September 2014.
Cover design by Gilles Vandenoostende.
Printed edition ISBN 978-91-981706-0-3

Author's email: martin@mitm.se
Comments and errata are welcome.
Spam, not so much.

Dedicated to Danielle, Charline, Milena, Julian, and Hania. You made this worth doing.

Martin Wehlou, 2014

"Anyone who is interested in the medical record systems of the future should read this book. Congratulations and thanks, Martin."

Ulf Jacobsson, founding partner of Mitt Hälsokonto AB, former CIO, Stockholm County Council.

"If there is a reference standard for the future design of the electronic healthcare record, this is the one."

Anders Westermark, MD.

"Famed conductor Leonard Bernstein composed his beautiful music while lying on a sofa. Archimedes had his flash of genius when reclining in a warm bath. And of course, a supine Michelangelo painted the Sistine Chapel. So after seeing your portrait on the cover of this book, I am convinced the content can be no less than paradigm shifting as it was clearly conceived during a state of blissful repose."

Fred Grazon, author of "The Lazy Way to Success".

"...I can't stop reading it. Much of the content, by all rights, should be a crushing bore, but it's not, in no small part due to your having revealed that the author is a living human with a sense of humor... congratulations on a superb piece of accessible technical writing."

Allen Cobb, author of "Brain Frieze", and sound artist.

Contents

Appendices

In a nutshell

If you're not sure if you want to invest the time or effort to read the whole book, this summary is for you.

Healthcare today is far from fulfilling its potential, and the reasons are numerous. One of the most important reasons is that the documentation system used today is fundamentally identical to the system used half a century ago, and it was known to be defective even then. Nothing much has been done to improve on it. The chance to improve it during the transition from paper records to electronic records was squandered.

There are two steps in the handling of every patient case: the diagnosis and the treatment. Both are very problematic and very much lacking in completeness, rigor, and consistency.

The first step, arriving at the right diagnosis, is usually a very haphazard process, relying on first impressions, intuition, and experience of the doctor. The potential solutions to the diagnostic problems have been thoroughly described by L. L. Weed [1], and again by Weed and Weed [2]. The book you are reading now, incorporates many of those findings and points, and adds to them in significant ways.

The second step, executing the right therapies and follow-up, has until now not been systematically analyzed and converted to a form amenable to automation and direct use by doctors. This analysis and how it should be implemented form the major part of this book.

Healthcare needs both these parts to exist, but they have to be built in such a way that they seamlessly integrate with each other and form a consistent whole. In what follows, it will be shown that these two steps can be integrated, but also that they enrich one another, and that together they form a whole that can be gradually introduced into a working healthcare system, while also being scalable. All the science and knowledge we've acquired means very little unless we

1

have tools to put that knowledge into practice, in a safe and consistent manner.

Doctors today are expected to keep the huge and ever changing knowledge base of medicine in their heads, performing both the complicated diagnostic and therapeutic procedures without any substantial knowledge-support systems. The only automation with any significant evolution is the documentation part, which, in comparison, has a relatively limited impact on the quality of diagnosis and care.

First, we need to make the initial data collection about the patient much more complete. This can best be done by using software to guide the gathering of symptoms and clinical signs.

Then we need to use the initial set of clinical data to make a complete list of possible diagnoses (or, as named in this book, "issues"). This candidate list of issues further informs us of clinical signs and tests that should be performed. This interaction between clinical findings and candidate issues continues until a small set of likely issues has been identified.

Each issue comes with a template that not only describes the diagnostic criteria for the issue, and thus informs the issue selection process, but also contains all the information needed for further investigations and therapies. This relieves the doctor from the hard and error-prone task of memorizing every possible therapy and its details.

The interaction of different issues in the same patient also becomes amenable to automated discovery and handling. All these features result in a change of the role of the doctor, from an unreliable source of memorized facts, to someone who, together with the patient, can judge and select among all the available diagnostic and therapeutic tools. The end result is a much higher consistency of care, and a reduction in errors of commission and omission.

A better document hierarchy that relates findings and conclusions to each other in the same way that the doctor actually reasons and decides, makes the documentation side of the EHR more amenable to understanding, and allows auditing of the record. At the same time, this structure solves several problems related to confidentiality and distribution of consistent parts of the medical record.

Introduction

The last couple of years I have been giving a lecture to the students of the "International Masters Program in Health Informatics" at the Karolinska Institute in Stockholm. Those lectures were based on a set of notes, and as time went by, I began to suspect that my notes harbored in them something bigger, maybe even a book. After some procrastination, I finally started expanding on them in January 2014, and what you see here is the result.

The target audience for the original notes consisted of students well-versed in both medicine and technology, which explains why the text tends to slide from one area into the other without much of a transition.

Converting these relatively limited notes to a full book implies that the target audience also changes in composition and character. Except for the aforementioned students, this includes doctors, nurses, and developers as intended audience. It is absolutely necessary that developers learn to appreciate the nuances of doctors' use of the medical record, while it is also essential that doctors learn to understand the technical limitations and possibilities inherent in these systems. Real solutions will not come from two or more professional groups working together, but will only come from each professional group reaching into the other's knowledge area and grabbing onto the stuff that they actually need. The design coherence needed for fully useful system designs must sprout from minds that can bridge the gap, and if these are in short supply, we must either produce more of them, utilize them better, or both.

Another very important point is this: don't look back! We have built IT systems based on how paper records work, and that didn't turn out well. We also have to stop looking at current systems for inspiration on how to build the next generation system, else they'll

3

also be dismal failures[1]. Forget about the past. Think up new systems from first principles, and it wouldn't even hurt if you assumed that every solution that looks most like what we have today is a bad idea and should be scrapped. The more different from that, the better.

There are also a number of evolutions in the development of the EHR that are worrisome. The structure of the medical records in their *current* form is often done to "make the computer understand" the healthcare process. If we think about the interaction of man and machine in healthcare, there are three possible ways to go:

- Man does his job and then feeds the machine data for safekeeping and management analysis purposes. This is what we have today for the main part.

- Man feeds the machine sufficiently understandable data, so that the machine can take the responsibility for the intellectual work. This is the road a number of systems, including OpenEHR, seem to take, even though there is no basis for thinking the machine can take over that job just yet. In the future, yes, but today?

- Man feeds the machine the minimum of data it needs to locate and gather the resources *man* needs to take responsibility for the intellectual work. This way we would improve man's ability to work correctly, while automating away man's main weaknesses, namely memorizing massive amounts of data, and consistent attention to detail. This is the way we must progress for the foreseeable future.

Far too few of the important angles have been the subject of objective research. It seems much of the field is built upon preconceived notions and assumptions by all involved, developers and medical staff alike, with mostly everyone assuming somebody else has it all figured out.

My (the author's) background, in brief, is in mathematics and medicine, including a residency in general, vascular, and thoracic surgery, and specialization in general medicine both in Belgium and Sweden. I've also developed software for more than 30 years in several domains, including medical applications. I'm still working part

---

[1] Yes, I take that as a given.

time in general practice and with clinical studies, while also writing software. Appendix B consists of an extended description of my background.

This book is organized in four parts:

Part I

The first part covers the major business cases for creating EHR systems. It also briefly analyzes what type of knowledge must be instilled into an individual to make her into a physician. A very quick recap of the history of medical records is then followed by a summary of the major ways the current EHR systems fail us.

Part II

We go into how current EHR systems work, and why they work as they do. It's hard to refrain from complaining about almost everything about these systems.

Part III

We look into how doctors work clinically, which real requirements we can derive from that, and how a correctly designed EHR system built on these requirements should look. We're making the assumption that the main goal of these systems should be to support clinical work, even though that is clearly not the case today. But it must be in the future.

Appendices

The last part contains one appendix that goes into more technical detail on the document-tree design. Unless you are into building systems, or comparing the designs in this book to other designs found elsewhere, you could probably safely skip this.

There is a second appendix with a longer history of the author's life story, at least as far as it applies to IT in medicine. This story does help explain at least some of the design choices made in the book.

In a text like this, one has to try to be clear with terminology. Here follow a few selected terms that have been raised to the level of "housebroken" and have been used as consistently as possible.

EHR

Electronic healthcare records (EHR) are often called "Electronic Medical Records" (EMR), and there seems to be no useful distinction between those two terms, even though there are arguments to the contrary [3]. If there is a difference then the "EMR" is more akin to the old paper records, while an "EHR" reaches beyond that to include both other organizations and other tools.

"EMR" occasionally means "Emergency Medical Responder", which can confuse things. It can also mean "Explosive Mishap Report", confusing things even further.

"EHR", on the other hand, has a much shorter list of interpretations. It does include "Explosive Hazards Reduction", which we can only see as a positive[1].

In this text, only the term "EHR" will be used, to the exclusion of "EMR" for the above reasons.

Issue

We need to have a name for the reason we see patients. We can't call it a "disease", since seeing a one-year-old for a regular developmental check isn't a "disease". We can't call it a "problem", since that can be insulting to the women we see for pregnancy follow-up. In this text, we will call these "issues", or sometimes "healthcare issues" for extra emphasis.

---

[1] See http://acronyms.thefreedictionary.com for more expansions on these abbreviations.

Issue Template

The management of a healthcare issue consists of a series of guidelines, references to publications, addresses we can refer to, a range of diagnostic techniques and therapeutic actions, advisories, medication types, products, dosages, equations, resource scoring, and more. This entire set of information and tools needed in the management of a healthcare issue is collected and organized into an "issue template". This term implies the technical implementation of the management of a healthcare issue, but here the term is used in both senses, as the collection of tools for management of an issue, and as the technical implementation of such a collection of tools.

Item

The term "item" is used in two senses. In the context of "issues", an "item" is a one-liner, a certain clinical finding with its set of possible values. It's the smallest part of a guideline, and therefore the constituent part for issue templates. For instance, "Blood pressure" can be an item, just as "Cardiac sounds" can be one.

In many other instances, "item" is used to mean what most people mean with "item". Such as "I have two items in a basket", or "are those two an item?"

His and hers

When writing a text, we always have the problem of what gender to use in third person. It's all too easy to write "him" all the time, and be revealed for the crypto chauvinists most of us older male doctors are deep down inside. But going to the other extreme, using "her" all the time, would lend a certain creepiness to the text. You can't go writing "him or her" everywhere either, since it simply looks ridiculous in the long run, and breaks the rhythm of the text, if it ever had one.

My chosen strategy is to mix it up a bit. In situations where I have to choose, I'll let the doctor be female, at least in situations where the doctor comes out looking smart. When the doctor is described as confused, or easily distracted, or of somewhat limited ability, I'll often use "him". Patients will usually be represented as males, too.

Yes, I realize this is also a prejudiced way of thinking and writing, but I'm less afraid of men than of women.

Acknowledgements

In no particular order, I'd like to thank the following people for constructive criticism and corrections of the text: Peter Olsson, Göran Agerberg, Johan Månflod, Jack Holleran, Ingrid Eckerman, Karin Lindhagen, and Anders Westermark.

Kim Nevelsteen contributed an enormous amount of high quality corrections to the text over an extended period of time.

Mary Brown of Capella University gave an insightful perspective on the US medical informatics scene.

Chris Bunch and Jeremy Dwight were kind enough to allow me to use the CHF guideline as an example, and both contributed important viewpoints on the creation and management of guidelines in general.

Bengt Dahlin contributed with his knowledge on the history of the medical record, which I made shamefully little use of. My bad.

I'd also like to thank Jerker Green and Ludwig Wänéus for many inspiring discussions on this theme.

A special thanks goes to Allen Cobb for making me think I should do this, for editorial help, and not least for getting me on the straight and narrow when it comes to using InDesign right.

And last, but not least, Hania Uscka-Wehlou, my wife, for inspiration, discussions, corrections, both linguistic and content-wise, LaTeX-assistance (for the drafts), and providing the encouragement to do this in the first place. And a lot of other things I'm not going to discuss here.

Part I

The basics

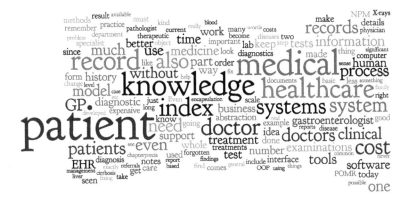

Summary

Before going into what's wrong with current systems, or how to build the next generation system, we have to review the basics of medical record keeping. These basics include identifying the driving business models, the stakeholders, the motivations of the stakeholders, and how doctors are trained and kept up to date. It must also include the history of the medical records, and an outline of the relationship between the medical record and the medical professional. In other words, how does the medical record actually help the medical professional do a better job?

CHAPTER 1

The business model

*What are the economic incentives for doing the right
thing? What is the "right" thing?*

There's a business model behind every decision on how to structure
healthcare and its support services. That business model could be
based on the overall cost to society of healthcare issues, versus the
cost of providing relief and prevention. These are the concerns at
a large scale, by region or nation. On a smaller scale, the business
model includes measures intended to reduce or displace costs, such
as moving them to other actors, and measures to optimize handling
of cases.

Let's take a few examples to illustrate the difference between the
large-scale business model and the small-scale business model.

Large-scale business model

If we calculate the cost to society of a case of polio, including treatment cost, assistance cost, and loss of productivity, we find that it's
much more expensive than the alternate cost of prevention [4]. It
should be obvious to anyone, except maybe to the anti-vaccination
nut cases, that global vaccination and ultimate eradication of the virus is an amazingly good idea.

The same calculation has also been made for certain types of cancer where we have useful screening methods—such as for breast
cancer, and colon cancer—and early detection and treatment is the
winning proposition, even without considering the human cost of
contracting cancer and having it detected too late for curative treatment.

We can also show that the correct and effective treatment of joint
disease, diabetes, hypertension, vascular disease, and a host of oth-

15

er problems, is a generally good idea from a national economics standpoint. All these things cost less to society as a whole if treated according to the state of the art. Even bleeding edge, and often extremely expensive, treatments are economically defensible once we take the evolution of the treatment into account over a period of time. Many of these initially expensive treatments lead to much more affordable and much more applicable treatments in the future; treatments that would never have been developed if the initial expense had not been made.

In short, paying for the best healthcare you can provide to your population is one hell of a good investment for any nation, even without considering the human cost of disease. No civilized nation would argue otherwise[1].

If healthcare is managed primarily according to the benefits to the nation as a whole, the systems developed for healthcare will focus on providing prevention and treatment from a medical perspective. The management of local expenditures will still play a role, but it will be a secondary role, since the calculation of "profit" makes no sense. There's no immediate and local payback for each treated patient; the payback is on a national scale and in a longer perspective.

Small-scale business model

The small-scale business model comes into play for a hospital, a department, or a practice. It's all the rage in models such as "New Public Management" (NPM), where departments are made into cost centers. Each department is incentivized to increase profits and reduce costs, on the assumption that if all departments become more cost conscious and more profitable, the organization, even the nation, as a whole benefits.

This model has been used for a long time in industry, and is becoming increasingly discredited even there, especially since the most profitable information technology companies are abandoning this model. Companies are increasingly seeing the benefit of having all departments work for the common good of the company as a whole, instead of artificially competing with one another. Healthcare seems to be a few decennia behind on this learning curve.

---

[1] Except the USA, but you guys are slowly getting the message, too.

When applying this cost center model to healthcare, at least in Sweden, a fictional cost is assigned to diagnostic and therapeutic actions. Medication prescribed is assigned a retail cost and "charged" to a fictional budget the prescribing organization has. Every radiology exam, or lab order, is similarly "charged" to the provider that ordered it. Every visit from a patient ends up on the "profit" side. The idea is that providers should be incentivized to save on costly examinations and treatments, while at the same time seeing as many patients as possible.

In this whole arrangement, two important incentives are missing. First, referrals are "free"; they don't incur a "charge" on the referrer. Secondly, there's no "reward" for actually making patients better. See where this is going?

In order to keep organizations in pretend money[2], the trick is to refer patients to someone else if it looks like their treatment is going to "cost" more than their visits bring in. On the other side of the referral, the referee is incentivized to refuse as many referrals as possible, especially if they look like they'll need a lot of expensive care. Or, alternatively, they're incentivized to only accept referrals where the originator of the referral has done as many expensive diagnostics as possible *before* referring the patient, on the referrer's own "dime". This turns the referring procedure into a confrontational game, instead of the cooperative effort to help and serve patients it should be.

Just to take an example: orthopedic surgeons take a lot of X-rays, since that is one of their most important diagnostic tools. They need them in most, but not all, patient cases. X-rays are therefore a large "cost" item in their budget, and they'd love to get patients referred who already had all the required X-rays taken beforehand to save on cost. In some places, they've taken this to the logical extreme. A department of orthopedics may not even accept a referral without accompanying X-rays. This causes a lot more X-rays than necessary to be made. The result is a hugely increased total cost of healthcare, unnecessary radiation exposure of patients, longer waiting times for other types of X-rays that are really necessary, and a loss for everybody's budget, *except* the department of orthopedics, which comes out looking more efficient.

---

[2] The departments with most pretend money left at the end of the year get preferential treatment when it comes to staffing and costs the year after.

Other examples are: the emergency department sending patients
to primary care for writing prescriptions, cardiologists referring patients back to the referrer with a recommendation for the referrer
to prescribe expensive medication the cardiologist prefers but can't
"afford", and more of that kind. In each instance, the patient is given
a run-around, while the *total* cost of care goes up, and the originator
of the problem is rewarded for being budget conscious. It's important to remember that the Swedish healthcare system is firmly "single
payer", so all these costs are ultimately covered by the same agency,
the state. The whole exercise is time-consuming, futile, idiotic, and
expensive.

If healthcare is provided under a small-scale business model such
as NPM, the supporting systems become essential to the process of
calculating and controlling costs, and keeping tabs on profitability,
for the department or institution using them. Any benefits on a national scale or long term will become invisible and ignored by the
local organization. This explains why there is *no business case* for
better healthcare under these ideologies, only for local sub-optimizations.

Small-business scale practices make sense in small businesses,
make very little sense in major corporations, and are absolutely toxic
to large-scale population concerns such as healthcare.

**Finally, we have to note that regardless of budgets, the
tax-paying citizens may want to pay for healthcare, even if it
isn't economically efficient. Human wellbeing consists of more
than financially measurable aspects of life. It's absurd to only invest in measures that result in a monetary return on investment.
If that were all we were concerned with as humans, we wouldn't
procreate.**

So, how come Swedish patients aren't worse off than they are?
With a model like the one just described, one would expect the
healthcare to be really crappy, but it isn't. The explanation for this
lies in a little bit of compensatory socialism; doctors aren't paid according to the outcome of the budget numbers, or the number of
patients. Doctors, in general, receive a fixed monthly salary, making
them largely insensitive to the NPM game. So even though it's a real
hassle having to argue with the orthopedics department and others
over referrals, doctors have no incentive to save on these fictional

charges, usually preferring to get the patient taken care of, regardless.

In short, it seems we're lucky that doctors don't need to care about the NPM numbers and budgets, partly neutralizing the best efforts of public management to corrupt and destroy the healthcare delivery process. One of two things can happen in the future: either the whole NPM idea is scrapped and replaced with a larger scale motivational system that measures and rewards healthcare outcomes, as it ought to do, or doctors move off the fixed salary regimen and become rewarded according to the NPM-based measurements, including small-scale monetary rewards. This would move Swedish healthcare to a similar system as the USA, almost certainly making healthcare as inefficient, and unequally distributed as it is there [5].

The stakeholders

A number of different professional groups have a stake in how the electronic healthcare record system works. Each of their primary uses of the system differs, and the demands on functionality are often in conflict.

Physicians mainly use current systems to record and retrieve patient histories, and to send and receive referrals. Other important uses are: the creation of prescriptions for medication, orders for radiology, orders for other technical diagnostic procedures, retrieval of radiology reports, and retrieval of lab reports. The system is also used to create correspondence, such as letters to patients.

A physician working in her own practice will also use the system to handle billing and payments.

The above reflects how current systems are used by doctors, but if the system was better, it could be used to provide support in the management of diagnosis and treatment of diseases, as well.

Nurses use the system to find out which diagnostics and treatments the physician has ordered, and to take notes on the progression and results.

Administrators mainly use the electronic healthcare record to measure the production as number of patients, severity of caseloads, how many beds are free, and more such. It is in administrators' interest that as much data as possible is coded in a way that allows statistical analysis of the organization and its throughput.

Since there are several stakeholders, all the groups should have their interests represented when designing the systems. As it is today, the interests of the management group not only overshadow the interests of the clinical groups, but are also increasingly displacing them. As a result, healthcare systems turn into management systems where the role of doctors and nurses, as far as the system is concerned, is progressively reduced to that of data-input clerks. There's very little, if any, effort to increase the utility of healthcare systems for better diagnostics and treatments.

CHAPTER 2

What are doctors made of?

How do we train doctors? How do we keep them
trained and sharp after that?

Naturally, we're all made of some calcium, water, neural cells, and not an inconsiderable amount of intestinal content, but what we really should discuss is what kind of knowledge and training is necessary to "build" a functioning physician. How do you go from being just a regular person to becoming a medical doctor able to make decisions affecting the health of a patient?

The knowledge we need can be divided into theoretical knowledge of the healthy human, knowledge about the mechanisms of disease, dexterity in clinical examinations, craftsmanship in diagnostic and therapeutic procedures, and current knowledge about diagnoses and therapies for a range of problems.

Theory of the healthy human

The initial courses at medical school are all focused on teaching the basic normal functioning of the human body. This includes stuff like biochemistry, anatomy, physiology, and more. As years go by and science advances, this body of knowledge tends to increase rather rapidly. We have long left behind us the time when an individual doctor could more or less have a grasp on all we know of the normal human body, so we have to assume that the practicing physician will only have at his fingertips the most rudimentary facts about the body. Any clinical work that requires a more detailed knowledge must also be supported by tools that provide the clinician with the knowledge needed.

Except for the occasional old anatomical atlas and well thumbed biochemistry book, you won't find many such tools in most clinician's offices, simply because very few of these tools exist. Even for the few that do exist, the clinician usually has just the one computer for the medical record, and those tools either don't work on that system, aren't allowed to be installed by less than helpful IT support staff, or don't work together with the existing medical-record software in any case.

Mechanisms of disease

Knowledge about mechanisms of disease is rapidly evolving. It's evolving so fast that any course knowledge the doctor may have is quickly outdated. There is a need for constant education about these developments, not on a yearly basis, but on a monthly or even weekly basis. Reading medical journals and participation in medical symposia also helps keep us updated, but it's a very hit-and-miss proposition if what is learned comes to practical use before it's forgotten again.

Clinical examinations

Clinical examinations include routines such as taking a blood pressure, listening to the chest sounds (and recognizing what you're hearing!), palpating the abdomen, testing reflexes, evaluating joints and tendons, and so on. *How* to do most of these clinical examinations must basically be taught in person, during classes or during work in the clinic with a real patient and a tutor. Some of these examinations can also usefully be taught to an already experienced physician with the aid of diagrams and explanations. An example can be seen in the excellent web pages from the American Academy of Family Physicians (AAFP [6]), about the examinations of the shoulder joint, a pretty complex subject (see Figure 2-1).

The illustration looks as if it came out of a jujitsu manual, but actually demonstrates one of the important clinical tests for instability of the shoulder joint. It is described in text, with an image illustrating how to perform the test, and the meaning of a positive test (anterior glenohumeral instability) is also mentioned briefly.

Anyone who is not a shoulder specialist would be hard pressed to remember this test, how it's done, and what it means. We've got

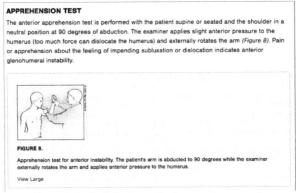

APPREHENSION TEST

The anterior apprehension test is performed with the patient supine or seated and the shoulder in a neutral position at 90 degrees of abduction. The examiner applies slight anterior pressure to the humerus (too much force can dislocate the humerus) and externally rotates the arm *(Figure 8)*. Pain or apprehension about the feeling of impending subluxation or dislocation indicates anterior glenohumeral instability.

FIGURE 8.

Apprehension test for anterior instability. The patient's arm is abducted to 90 degrees while the examiner externally rotates the arm and applies anterior pressure to the humerus.

View Large

Figure 2-1. A clinical examination, as shown on the AAFP.org site.

hundreds of other clinical tests to remember, and this is one of those that are easily forgotten if not done regularly.

What we need in practice is a quick reference that pops up when we have a patient with shoulder problems. That reference should include this and other relevant tests, so we know what to do. As it is today, doctors have to know about the existence of the AAFP website, know where to look and go find the test. Not only that, we will also have to describe the test, at least briefly, in the medical record together with the result. If we don't, a future reader of the patient record will either not know what we're talking about, or will have to look up the test and the meaning anew, and this process will have to be repeated each time the record is read.

Clearly, what we need is a direct and current link between the documentation for how the test is done, with the result of performing the test on the patient, and have all that become a part of the patient's medical record[1].

Craftsmanship

Craftsmanship comes into play when it's time to draw blood, open the abdomen, hack off limbs, check the eyesight or retina, or aspirate earwax. Depending on specialty, this craftsmanship can go from the

---

[1] Spoiler alert: the solution is an iotaMed-type application, as I describe in the chapter "The issue oriented record" on page 125 and onward.

very limited, as for psychiatrists[2], to the very extensive, as for surgeons.

Most, if not all, of this craftsmanship must be learned the same way iron smiths learn their skills, in a master-apprentice arrangement. When these skills need updating, doctors again go watch each other do whatever it is that is being done, then try it themselves under initial supervision. There is some help that IT systems could provide for this process, but nothing earth-shaking[3]. This type of learning process probably needs to stay the way it is for the foreseeable future.

Diagnostic and therapeutic knowledge

Knowledge about diagnostic tools falls partly into the same category as "clinical examinations", but it encompasses much more. Knowing which radiology studies to order for confirmation of exactly which diseases, is a skill that needs constant updating. Knowing which lab tests are available and what they mean, also takes some considerable work to keep up to date. Even knowing which diseases *can* be diagnosed using available tools is far from simple. Worse yet, even knowing which diseases *exist* is a challenge[4].

The therapeutic arsenal, i.e. the number and kind of methods we have at our disposal to alleviate diseases, is changing at a fantastic pace. There is no way a practicing physician can keep track of even a fraction of what is going on in this area, except for a tiny part of a single specialty. Even knowing which other specialty to refer a patient to, or even that the patient should be referred at all, is complicated enough to be regarded as a significant problem in its own right.

The sum total of all diagnostic and therapeutic knowledge is so vast, and so rapidly changing and expanding, that it's impossible to rely on human memory alone. There are not enough hours in a day

---

[2] Most of a psychiatrist's skills lie in other areas than the purely manual.

[3] There's a lot of hay being made of computer simulations for training surgeons, but it's out of proportion to its relative importance, at least compared to other urgent problems in medicine that need computerization. But there's more money to be made more quickly selling simulators, or—just as likely—it's easier for journalists to understand.

[4] Which, by the way, is far fewer than the internet would have you believe.

for any doctor to even barely keep up. This is where we need knowledge-based tools the most. But to make them even remotely useful, they have to be linked to the medical record in such a way that searches are triggered and enhanced based on the information about the patient in the records, and that the results from such searches also become part of the patient's information, including the conclusions the doctor drew from the searches in view of the patient's particulars.

Having searches of the universe of knowledge unconnected to the patient record not only increases the cognitive load on the doctor beyond the bearable, but also loses a large part of the advantage of automation, since the relationships found, and decisions made by the doctor, cannot be persisted into the record. This implies they can't be used as a base for future analysis and decisions. The waste of human intellectual effort is simply epic.

CHAPTER 3

Encapsulation

*Why do we need specializations? How do we keep
them independent enough to evolve?*

If we forget about healthcare for a minute, and look at how information is handled in other parts of science and society, we can see that as the information and knowledge volume increases, delegation compensates for complexity and allows us to keep evolving. As an example that should be easy to visualize, let's take programming.

Without going into the entire history of computing, we can claim with confidence that one of the most important steps in the evolution to highly complex systems was the invention of object-oriented programming (OOP). OOP is based on the following ideas:

- The details of an implementation should remain invisible to everyone using an object in a larger context, so much so that the internal coding, the implementation, can change as long as the use of it by other objects does not change.

- The interface to the object should be minimal and contain nothing that depends on the exact inner workings of the object.

- At each level of abstraction, the programmer composes objects and creates a new object with a higher level of abstraction.

This way, OOP leads to ever higher levels of abstraction, each level being free from knowledge of details of objects at lower levels of abstraction.

Correctly done, OOP removes from view all the internal complexity you don't need at any particular level of abstraction. This staged reduction of detail, opaque encapsulation, is what turns a potentially exponential growth of detail into a linear process that can be handled by human minds.

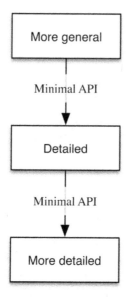

Figure 3-1. Encapsulation flow.

In medicine, the same process applies. The patient talks to the general practitioner (GP) using a high-level API: *"I'm sick. I think it's my liver. It runs in the family."*

The GP reasons to himself in much more detail: *"The liver. Right... What he probably means is that he's prone to nausea and stomach aches, but that's probably because his whole family is living off hamburgers and get into drunken fist fights over the TV remote. Anyhow, I'll check his transaminases, not forgetting the gamma-GT."* But what he says to the patient after poking his abdomen for a bit is something like: *"Umm... your liver is maybe a little tender, we'll run some tests."*

If the GP had gone to a continuing professional education[1] class and learned that there is now a virus causing a deadly disease involving symptoms of nausea, fights, and remotes, and that it was brought to earth by the moon landing crew[2], he would still have responded the same way: *"We'll run some tests"*. In other words, the change in the GP's internal implementation of how to do medicine in a family

---

[1] Continuing Professional Education (CPE). The ongoing refresher courses intended to keep professionals up to date.

[2] Don't worry, I'm lying.

practice in the space age does not lead to a change in his information interface towards the patient. The GP is fully encapsulated and OOP compliant.

Let's push this example a bit and assume something is terribly wrong with the lab tests and the GP refers the patient to a gastro-enterologist with the general question: *"What's up with this liver? Maybe a biopsy would be a good idea?"*

Now, let's further assume that the gastroenterologist agrees[3], goes on to make an appointment for a biopsy, chooses the most suitable ultrasound transducer, the right needle gauge and length, etc, and does the biopsy. The gastroenterologist, in turn, sends off the specimens to a pathologist for microscopic, and possibly histochemical, analysis.

The pathologist also does his thing coloring, embedding, slicing and dicing, and all this results in an answer from the pathologist to the gastroenterologist detailing the microscopic findings and elaborating on the type of tissue damage seen. The terms "cirrhosis" and "steatosis" may be used in this report. A few other minor types of cell damage or proliferation are also noted. Since the pathologist does not report all the different preparation steps or solutions and equipment used, the pathologist is also encapsulated and has a restricted interface versus the gastroenterologist.

The gastroenterologist looks at this report, decides from the clinical picture and the pathology report that the cirrhosis is significant, the steatosis less so—it's very common in the general population— and that the other findings of minor cell damage are coincidental and irrelevant for the current major complaints. So the gastroenterologist reports only the most significant findings to the GP and just takes notes of the less significant findings in his own notes, just in case they will turn out to be relevant later.

So, in summary, the gastroenterologist reports to the GP something like this: *"The biopsy showed a moderate degree of cirrhosis with some steatosis"*.

At this point, the GP is supposed to understand "cirrhosis" and "steatosis", and more or less know what to do about it (cut out the alcohol and the hamburgers; the fist fights present no problem). But the GP does not need to know how to do a liver biopsy or how to prepare the samples for microscopy or even how cirrhosis looks in a mi-

---

[3] This does happen.

croscope. Even if the specialist buys new equipment and then does his biopsies in a different and better way, this makes no difference in the interface between the GP and the specialist. In this example, the gastroenterologist is fully encapsulated versus the GP.

This encapsulation allows functionality at every layer of abstraction to evolve independently. The GP can change and improve his methods without the patient noticing[4]. The gastroenterologist can change and improve his methods without changing his interface towards the GP, and the pathologist can modify his methods without changing his interface towards the gastroenterologist. This is the only way to allow medicine to evolve, going from the "super GP" who knew all of medicine in the middle ages[5] to the super specialists of today.

It is relatively easy to see that the same process of layered levels of abstraction of knowledge applies in all intellectual human endeavors, not only programming and medicine.

And here comes the moral of this story:

To allow medicine to work efficiently, we must mirror the same levels of abstraction, encapsulation, and separation of concerns in the EHR as the EHR becomes our primary tool. Only high-level information should be shared by default, not the details. If we keep flattening the EHR as is generally done today, with access to every detail at every level, we're moving medicine back into the middle ages instead of forwards into the 21st century.

And, more bluntly:

Large, unified EHR systems are a really bad idea. A much better idea is loosely coupled specialist systems, each with a narrow interface, mirroring object-oriented systems and allowing full knowledge encapsulation.

Exercise for the student: how does this destroy the idea of allowing the patient access to the EHR as it is implemented today?

---

[4] Except as better, quicker, and perhaps even more gratifying encounters with primary care.

[5] Which wasn't much.

CHAPTER 4

The history of medical records

*We have to know where we came from to understand
how we arrived where we are now.*

As in all books, there is this "history" thing. But in this case, the history is essential to understanding why things are as bad as they are.

(In what follows, remember that I'm old enough to have actually lived through the described evolutionary stages myself, and I ain't dead yet.)

The absence of records

Not long ago, some family practitioners had no medical records at all. When I first took over a practice in Belgium in the 80's, the "records" I got consisted of two stacks[1] of documents:

1. Letters, lab reports, and other documents that my predecessor had not yet seen and discussed with the patient, in reverse chronological order. In other words, they were dumped on top of each other as they came in.

2. The same kind of documents, after they'd been seen, in order of their processing. In other words, they were dumped on top of each other in the second heap once seen and discussed with the patient.

The system, if you can call it that, worked as follows: the patient came in and asked what the specialist said or what the blood tests showed. The doctor then asked the patient at approximately what

---

[1] Literally stacks: one of them was a meter high, the other a third of that.

date the visit to the specialist occurred or the drawing of blood, then
proceeded to locate the document in stack number one. After reading
it and discussing it with the patient, he prescribed something or other and off the patient went. The document ended up on stack number two and was never read again. The whole incident then lodged
somewhat loosely in the memory of the doctor and hopefully more
permanently in the memory of the patient.

Obviously, this "system" can only work for a limited number of
patients, and only if they stay with the same doctor for a long time.
This kind of patient-doctor relationship was common back then, but
was rapidly becoming extinct as both doctors and patients became
much more mobile. Also, the number of doctors, both general practitioners and specialists involved in the care of a patient, is increasing,
resulting in the number of contacts between each doctor and any
particular patient going down.

But the worst aspect of this old type of doctor-patient relationship is that it is dangerous. Important details are forgotten, and the
patient's history can't effectively be transferred from one doctor to
his successor.

Paper-based mementos

Obviously, this was a terrible state of affairs. Around this time, most
GPs in Belgium started keeping a real medical record for two reasons:

1. Fear of lawsuits. If you're sued for malpractice and you have no
    records at all, you're pretty much doomed.

2. To memorize details, such as exactly which medicine was pre-
    scribed for exactly what period of time, dosage, and exactly
    when, and blood pressure measurements, and such.

In other words, the paper record evolved to store hard to remember
details in diagnosis and treatment on the one hand, and simultaneously to be a log of all interactions with the patient for legal reasons.
The knowledge about the patient as such, his diseases, preferences,
and most of all the overall plan in the diagnosis and treatment, was
not so much written down as memorized by the doctor. After all,

the patient always went to the same doctor anyway, so why write it down?[2]

Sweden had proper records for patients much earlier than Belgium. General practitioners ("provincial doctors") had an obligation to keep notes on both patients and events in the environment, and this started roughly 200 years ago. They had to report yearly to the authorities on the state of health and risk factors in their regions. About a hundred years ago, there were already regulations about the minimum content of medical patient records, but not on their form. Most records were extremely brief, and most information about the patient was never written down, but maintained in the head of the doctor. Even as late as 50 years ago, most records were kept on index cards, since that provided ample space for the amount of information actually kept on a patient.

In the 1970's, it became more common to have several doctors managing the same patients, so more extensive records were needed. A Swedish standard form of medical records was developed (the Spri project [7]), and a number of elements of the records became well defined.

The problem-oriented medical record (POMR)[3] was introduced in the 1970's. As part of POMR, the subjective-objective-assessment-planning (SOAP) model for the record was introduced. The SOAP model, without the underlying POMR model, can be seen in widespread use in other parts of Europe, but is fairly uncommon in its pure form in Sweden today.

During the 1980's, computers came into medical practice on a large scale. The applications were largely based on the preexisting paper records and were in fact treated as a quicker and more advanced carrier of the same basic information. It was never conceived as anything more than a record that allowed efficient retrieval of essentially the same information as had previously been kept on paper and in folders and cabinets.

A very good source for much more detailed information on the history, the structure, the events, and the systems (in Swedish), can be found on Bengt Dahlin's site [9].

---

[2] It was also a great incentive for the patient to stick to the same doctor.

[3] The problem-oriented medical record was described by Lawrence L. Weed in his book published in 1970 [1]. A summary of the idea can be found at The Free Dictionary [8].

The key thing to remember is this:

The classic paper-based medical record was only intended to support the family doctor in the maintenance of hard to memorize details and was never designed to contain the overall picture of the patient or any diagnostic or therapeutic plan. Since there is no assigned and permanent doctor in most practices anymore, it makes no sense to automate the paper-based records without considerable adaptation to the new medium. But that is exactly what has happened. The electronic record is designed as if it was a paper record, but in digital form. All the opportunities for improvements that the digital form brings have been squandered. Current medical records are characterized by a torrent of largely useless details without a unifying context.

CHAPTER 5

How should the EHR assist us?

*As a doctor, what help do I expect from a well-de-
signed medical system? And why am I not getting it?*

It's useful to compare the tools and methods we use in medicine with
how other professions evolved. All professions have in common that
they use knowledge, methods, and tools to achieve a goal. Medicine
is more lopsided than most professions, lacking many of the tools
we need for optimal performance. Not so coincidentally, it is unique
in the sense that most tools for medical professionals are specified,
designed and developed by lay people, while most other professions
are not so unfortunate. Pilots have a say in how cockpits should look,
architects have influence on the software they use for design, but
doctors often get medical-record software that no doctor would have
specified. The result is a system with entire missing areas of coverage, and we need to look into what those missing areas are.

Compare to other knowledge areas

We should not have to make a choice between a system that assists
us in decision making and a system that documents our actions, since
the very process of working through a problem using knowledge
support can be automatically documented, and in itself covers a major part of that documentation.

There is information, such as the patient history, that is not structured and not a part of a process. This information is not an explicit
part of any decision tree, but is very important when it comes to the
consideration of the selection of the overall approach to the issue,
which is a discussion between doctor and patient, where the patient's
choices come first. At the same time, these unstructured notes cannot
be directly used in the decision process for any particular issue.

With this reasoning, we arrive at the conclusion that any other free-form medical-record notes are a symptom of defective knowledge-support functionality, which is a good description of *all* of our notes the way they are done currently, since there is no knowledge-support functionality at all worth the name in any of our systems.

To see how the EHR fails in assisting doctors in their work, we

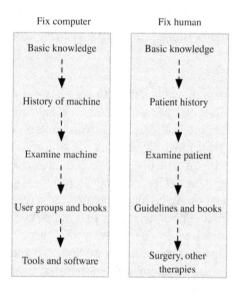

Figure 5-1. Comparing how to fix two similarly complex things.

need to compare it to other known processes that do work much better, and the example chosen here is "fixing a computer", since that is what most of us do far too often.

If we put the process of "fixing a computer" right next to the process of "fixing a human", we can find the same five stages or phases in both processes (see Figure 5-1).

The first part, "basic knowledge" (of computers), has the corresponding "basic knowledge" (of humans) in the other column. These requirements are somewhat analogous for the two knowledge areas.

The second step, the "history" part, is the only thing we have developed to a significant extent in EHR systems. Similar to the "computer fixing" process, this is not the most important step. It's nice to have, sure, but surprisingly easy to live without.

When we get to step three, "examine machine" vs "examine human", we find support for some, such as radiology, lab, and most therapies, in the EHR.

The real "meat" of the process to fix a computer is in the fourth step: "user groups and books". Not many computers would be fixed today without the ability to reference what other people have seen and how to fix it (or not, as may be). Trying to fix a computer without any reference to these resources is doomed to failure except in the most trivial cases.

Actually, the same is true for medicine. Since we don't have the same kind of easily available resources, medical practice is still in the 1980's if we compare it to fixing computers. We're still off-line, so to speak. We can fix humans, but the only knowledge we can use is what was hammered into us at medical school, or that we can fortuitously remember from a more recent CPE class.

That fourth step, the step that really makes a difference, is all about gathering recent knowledge about a problem and its solution. That part is missing entirely in the EHR systems we have today. Yes, those resources are available elsewhere, but they are both hard to locate and hard to use *while examining and treating a patient*, the very time when these tools could make the most difference.

Let's make another comparison: the architect's productivity has certainly increased with the introduction of email and software that allows him to both write and maintain textual documentation, but the real advance of architecture is enabled by computer-aided design software. Where is the computer-aided design software equivalent for medicine?

Since most current EHR systems are specified by civil servants, it's only natural that any requirements for providing better healthcare, quicker diagnostics and more consistent therapies have been left out entirely. None of these things matter to the administrators, so they simply don't care to specify any such functionality.

You get what you pay for, or rather, you get what he who pays for it asks for. And healthcare functionality is not a part of that.

The questions it should answer

Building on the example in the previous section, we can translate that into a few different ways the software should help us.

What should I do?

The first thing the software should help me with is a guideline on basic stuff, such as:

- What history elements must I query the patient about?

- Which clinical signs and examinations are basic to most problems and should be considered[1]?

If I have a working hypothesis, the software should present me with signs and techniques that can be helpful to confirm or exclude that hypothesis. It should also present the major criteria for a diagnosis, without drawing any conclusions automatically. For more on this, see the chapter "How active should the software be?" on page 121.

How should I do it?

When I do a clinical examination or determine clinical signs, the software should:

- List the signs and examinations related to this, their names and a list of possible outcomes.

- Give me an informational page showing me how to perform the clinical examination.

- Give me information about what the clinical examination results mean and imply. Included here should be pointers to other examinations that could be valuable to complement the result.

---

[1] "Considered" means just that; you should think about it, and do it if you think you must. The point here is that if you don't do something in a guideline, it should be because you had a reason not to do it, not that you simply forgot.

If I decide to order a diagnostic test in the form of lab tests or technical diagnostics such as X-ray or ultrasound, the software should assist me as follows:

- Show which diagnostics are available.

- Show what prerequisites apply to the diagnostics, and when they shouldn't be performed (contra-indications).

- Show the relative cost of the diagnostic, both in resource use and in costs to the patient (radiation load, pain, risk for complications, time, etc).

- Show where the test can be done, and what provider to send the order to.

- Help me fill in a form for ordering the test, including all the elements the intended recipient of the form has determined is needed for the order.

- Helpfully propose the right documents from the records to include with the referral.

What did I forget?

The application should point out to me what I forgot, such as:

- Which other diagnoses should I consider and exclude for this patient? That is, present me with a list of "differential diagnoses"[2].

- Which lab tests or diagnostic tests have I forgotten to perform to confirm this tentative diagnosis?

- Which therapy have I forgotten to start, or stop, for this diagnosis?

- Which reporting have I forgotten to perform?

---

[2] A "differential diagnoses" are the result of the process whereby we look for alternative diagnoses, that is, other explanations. Most findings can have a multitude of explanations.

As before, the system shouldn't tell me what to do, only what to *consider*. As a user, I should feel comfortable that I've considered all the angles and that my choices are made not from ignorance or happenstance, but from weighted judgment of all the elements.

History in context

When retrieving the history of the patient, the EHR system should present a list of issues for the patient, and all notes, conclusions, examinations, and other documents *in the context of their respective issue*.

Any notes, conclusions, or findings relevant to more than one issue should be presented in the context of *all* those issues.

CHAPTER 6

Conclusion

In the first part of this book, we went over *why* current EHR systems were built, and the financial motivations and thinking behind them. We also touched on *who* has a stake in these systems. The reason we need to know about the *why* and the *who* is that these factors largely determine how the systems are built. If we want to change how they are built, we need to understand—and change!—the motivations and incentives of the people making the decisions.

We also worked through the other components of the problem, namely the training and source of reference knowledge for the working physician, in an effort to clarify what support the doctor may need in her work. Is the training adapted to a society with capable computing support, and is that computing support designed to effectively enhance the doctor's abilities?

Lastly, we summarized the support doctors need at the highest, simplest possible level of abstraction.

In the next part, we'll show how current systems work (or don't work, as may be).

Part II

Current systems

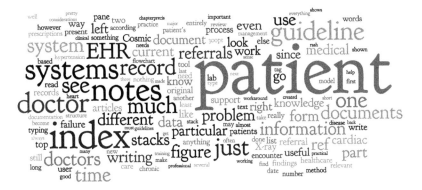

Summary

In these chapters, you will find an example of a current electronic healthcare record system, and how we work with it. We'll also describe which knowledge-support systems are available today and make a few points about their usefulness, or lack thereof, and try to identify what is missing to make them more useful.

We'll also analyze how a doctor works, and how she interacts with the electronic healthcare record, including the limitations due to time and place of use.

Finally, we'll go into the information model that is used in current systems, and what's wrong with it.

This part is mainly catering to the non-physician reader, providing the background necessary to understand why our current systems don't satisfy the real needs of doctors, and by implication, what needs to change. Doctors are also encouraged to read these chapters to see the assumptions and the background the author had when writing this text. Contexts vary, and yours may be different.

CHAPTER 7

The goal of the system

What seems to be the goal of current systems? Are we happy with how that turned out?

The goal of the system should be to help the healthcare professional do a better job. Some functions of EHR systems support data entry and communication; functions which are generally fairly well developed in current systems. What is almost entirely lacking, however, is knowledge and process support, as described in the chapter "How should the EHR assist us?" on page 35. Some simpler processes for nursing can be found here and there, but nothing really significant is going on in this space.

Note well: of course there are knowledge- and process-support initiatives out there, but there are no significant such initiatives that are fully a part of the EHR. There's a great number of such stand-alone initiatives, fragmented and each covering just a part of the problem area. But even if there were wall-to-wall coverage in such a tool, it's still not a part of the healthcare documentation process. If you have to interrupt the regular documentation process to go look up something, and what you find does not automatically become documented, it's not only harder to do, it also does not enrich the documentation with any reasoning resulting from the knowledge you looked up. It's not sufficient to define in the documentation what you do to the patient, it's essential that you document *why*, or *why not*, you are doing it, and that motivation is lacking if the knowledge support is not integrated into the same tool as the documentation.

One could argue that the EHR has only a documenting function, and that the knowledge-support function should be separately implemented and provided, but that would by necessity imply duplication of effort and redundant information. One could also argue, as this book does, that the EHR has erroneously been viewed and developed

47

as a documenting tool instead of a supporting tool. Current systems are also increasingly subverted to become data gathering tools for management purposes *instead* of a tool for healthcare provision, largely due to a power grab of administrators in healthcare.

A nice illustration of how badly current systems are conceived, at least from a practical healthcare perspective, came in a New York Times article celebrating the joy of having *someone else* update the EHR:

> "Without much fanfare or planning, scribes have entered the scene in hundreds of clinics and emergency rooms. Physicians who use them say they feel liberated from the constant note-taking that modern electronic health records systems demand. Indeed, many of those doctors say that scribes have helped restore joy in the practice of medicine, which has been transformed—for good and for bad—by digital record-keeping." [10]

If you introduce a new IT system to help a particular professional do a better job, and one of the most celebrated advances in the use of that IT system is having someone else manage it so you don't have to come into contact with it, your system is pretty much condemned as nothing but a drag on the user. It's hard to think up a more damning verdict than that.

CHAPTER 8

Legacy EHR example: Cosmic

To show what the problem is, let's deconstruct a typical current EHR system.

We'll illustrate how current systems work by using examples from Cambio Cosmic, a system the author has used quite a bit. The descriptions and screen shots aren't of the most recent version and some improvements have been made since these were taken[1], but fundamentally, it's still working according to the same principles. It's important to stress that Cosmic is certainly not the worst system out there; it could conceivably even be the best. But it is definitely representative of the sorry state of systems we have.

In the first screen shot (Figure 8-1) we see a window showing the notes for the current patient. At the top of the screen we have the demographics, showing the personal number and name of the patient (a fake test patient). The top right shows three buttons in different colors indicating different kinds of warnings.

The right large pane shows the contents of notes selected from the left pane.

The left pane lets you select what to show in the right pane. It's a list of sources of documentation, typically different departments within primary care or hospital care. It's basically an organizational chart.

County-owned primary care is one section, while privately-owned primary care centers have their own sections. Each specialty department, such as "urology" and "orthopedics", is grouped under a larger umbrella (such as "surgery"). This must be wonderful for a civil servant to see, but is pretty much pointless to the work of a doctor. Yes, we do *occasionally* want to know *where* the patient has been,

---

[1] I would like to use more recent screen shots, but I very much doubt they'd let me take them.

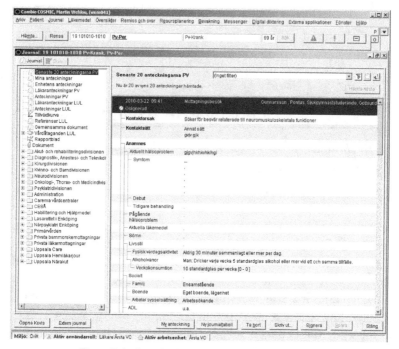

Figure 8-1. Cosmic, viewing the notes in the record.

but generally we're much more interested in *what* and *why*, which this list doesn't help with at all.

This left pane is a fantastic illustration of what's wrong with current systems. It's pretty clear it was designed, or at least specified, by a lay person *imagining* what he would like to see there if he were a doctor, and then forcing doctors to see just that. It's very doubtful that a doctor would have chosen that view to occupy such a dominating part of the work-flow, if given a free choice.

If you look at the top of the left pane in Figure 8-1, you'll see two tabs. The left one says "Journal" ("Notes"), while the right one says "Skriv" ("Write"). This is where you switch both panes over from reading to writing.

When in writing mode, the left pane changes to show all the "keywords" (subtitles), you can enter information into (see Figure 8-2). Whatever you write in the right pane is entered into the field contents of the keyword you have selected on the left. At the top, above the entry field in the right pane, you can select date, time, contact (encounter), and where you are. Again, in this screen, you see an em-

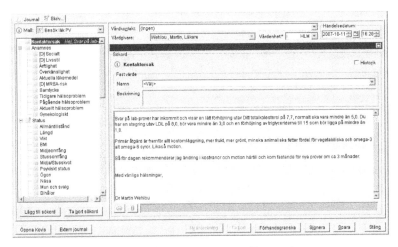

Figure 8-2. Cosmic in notes-writing mode.

phasis on "who", "where", and "when", but not so much on "what" and "why", which would be more useful.

What we also see is a structure determined by those keywords to the left. This neatly shows what the developers have understood when we say "structured records", namely a text divided into sections according to some fairly random list of different terms. That's not what most doctors would regard as a medically sensible structure, however. Anyone can slice any text any number of ways without improving its utility, as we witness here. The "structure" we'd like to see is a division into diagnostic plans, intentions, deductions, findings, and the underpinnings of those. There's nothing of that in Cosmic, or in any other current EHR systems.

While we create a prescription in Cosmic, the screen looks like in Figure 8-3. The entire working space on the screen is occupied by all the stuff you need to prescribe a medication. The only other things that still appear are my name, the patient's name[2], and the contact date and time. That's it. It's obvious that the developers didn't see that prescriptions have anything to do with notes, referrals, lab, or just about anything else in the records, or that the doctor would need to refer to anything else while creating prescriptions. With this setup, you can't. When seeing a patient for hypertension, for instance, it's as easy (or difficult) to prescribe a blood pressure lowering medication as it is to prescribe the pill, or morphine, or a drug against Par-

---

[2] Fictional, of course.

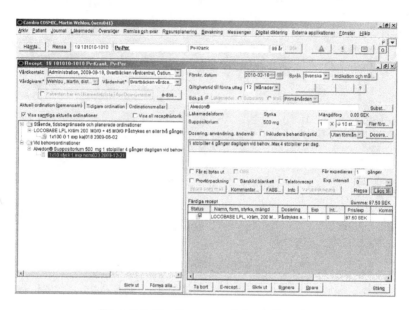

Figure 8-3. Creating a prescription in Cosmic.

kinson's disease. The system is totally oblivious to what disease is being managed. It doesn't help and it doesn't hinder (too much). If I send a referral, likewise the system allows me, with exactly the same level of support or hindrance, to send it to a cardiologist, a kidney specialist, or, why not, a psychiatrist, or a hearing aid service. It has no preferences and is completely insensitive to the medical context.

If you had created a system for photographers with this attitude and domain implementation, it would contain functions for finding models, taking pictures, developing film, making copies, and invoicing clients, flushing toilets, and clearing gutters, but the picture taking would have no relationship to either models or film, the development task would involve bottles of solutions, but no film or copies, while the invoicing would have no relationship to anything else, making it as easy to invoice a photo shoot as a dozen dead rabbits. No photographer in his right mind would buy an application like that.

There's no screen shot here of how you write referrals with Cosmic, but you're not missing much. It's the same kind of thing, where once you start writing, you see nothing else, and cannot look up anything else. The referral itself is not connected to any particular disease or other documents, and is, for all practical purposes, as integrated into the patient's narrative as a dozen dead rabbits.

It bears repeating: *Cosmic isn't worse than anything else out there, it may even be the best system of them all. It's probably pretty much representative of the current market.* Which, when you think of it, isn't a very comforting thought.

CHAPTER 9

Knowledge support

What kind of knowledge support do we have today?
Do we use it? If not, why?

As doctors or nurses, we can't possibly keep everything we should know just in our heads. And even if we could, things change as science advances. There is such an enormous amount of data we have to make use of, and an ever growing avalanche of new findings. There's no way we can drink from this fire-hose and do real work at the same time.

Depending on how fresh the information is, and the level of detail, it is available as original articles, review articles, textbooks, guidelines, and/or as CPE course material.

Original articles

According to the Medline Fact Sheet [11], there are more than 19 million references to original articles in their database. Another 2,000 - 4,000 are added *daily*. Even though everything we need to know in our daily practice is in there *somewhere*[1], this information isn't useful in clinical practice in its raw form. Researchers working on a particular topic have great use of this resource, but for a clinician having a patient in her office, it's practically useless. You can't just say to the patient: *"I have to go read up on your problem for a bit. Grab a coffee, and I'll be back in a couple of weeks."*[2]

---

[1] This glosses over the practical techniques, the judgement, and the experience we need as doctors, focusing solely on the scientific findings.

[2] Well, strictly speaking you can, but the patient will be gone by the time you get back.

At times, publications containing remarkable and important discoveries are widely read by doctors, but this is just an infinitesimally small fraction of the total published mountain of articles. And we can't just ignore the rest. Most of them form the basis of future diagnostic and therapeutic principles, so we have to use a system to reduce them to a more digestible form.

Review articles

Well-informed authors regularly write reviews of the most important papers in their field and publish those in the same type of medical journals where the original papers are usually published. These review articles allow non-specialist doctors to get a good overview of a particular subject and the current state of knowledge about it. While writing these reviews, the authors use their best judgment to sift through the underlying original articles to bring forward the most relevant and trustworthy findings, so the rest of us don't have to do that.

These review articles are still too detailed and specialized to be directly useful in patient care in general, but are often just fine as a tool to keep up in a field in which the doctor sees a lot of patients, but not necessarily does research.

Textbooks

Textbooks constitute the next level up, and the quality of the information is similar to reviews, but as a collection of related subjects for a certain medical specialty.

While original articles and review articles presume the reader is already familiar with the subject, the textbook does not, and starts from basics. Textbooks are rarely useful for a practicing doctor, except as a reminder of what she learned in medical school. Additionally, textbooks are much too expensive to buy just to keep up with the science. They're also not updated timely enough for that use.

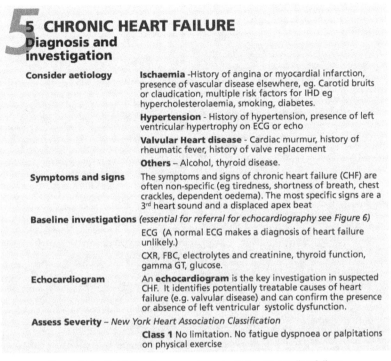

5 CHRONIC HEART FAILURE
Diagnosis and investigation

Consider aetiology	**Ischaemia** -History of angina or myocardial infarction, presence of vascular disease elsewhere, eg. Carotid bruits or claudication, multiple risk factors for IHD eg hypercholesterolaemia, smoking, diabetes.
	Hypertension - History of hypertension, presence of left ventricular hypertrophy on ECG or echo
	Valvular Heart disease - Cardiac murmur, history of rheumatic fever, history of valve replacement
	Others – Alcohol, thyroid disease.
Symptoms and signs	The symptoms and signs of chronic heart failure (CHF) are often non-specific (eg tiredness, shortness of breath, chest crackles, dependent oedema). The most specific signs are a 3rd heart sound and a displaced apex beat
Baseline investigations *(essential for referral for echocardiography see Figure 6)*	
	ECG (A normal ECG makes a diagnosis of heart failure unlikely.)
	CXR, FBC, electrolytes and creatinine, thyroid function, gamma GT, glucose.
Echocardiogram	An **echocardiogram** is the key investigation in suspected CHF. It identifies potentially treatable causes of heart failure (e.g. valvular disease) and can confirm the presence or absence of left ventricular systolic dysfunction.
Assess Severity – *New York Heart Association Classification*	
	Class 1 No limitation. No fatigue dyspnoea or palpitations on physical exercise

Figure 9-1. Guideline for management of chronic cardiac failure, diagnosis and investigation.

Guidelines

Guidelines are based on original research and reviews, and turn that content into practical use advice. If there's a study that says it's advantageous to the patient to apply therapy X, the guideline recommends therapy X, at least if it's available in the relevant region.

In theory, guidelines are entirely based on science, the interest of the patient, and the resources available, and are short and sweet enough that they can be read, understood, and applied while the patient is present. In practice, however, these guidelines are often influenced by considerations that have nothing to do with the patient's immediate interest, but by political and economic incentives. If those economic considerations are of the kind that optimizes healthcare in a larger perspective, it's reasonable to accept that, but manipulative bureaucrats sometimes compromise the integrity of these motives to such a degree that guidelines are getting a bad rap as being a tool for civil servants to control medical professionals, rather than a tool to improve the qual-

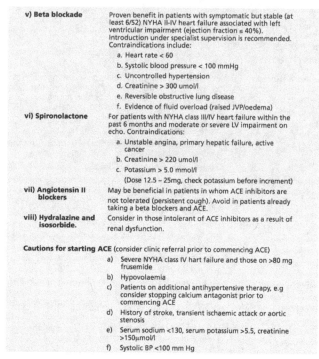

v) Beta blockade	Proven benefit in patients with symptomatic but stable (at least 6/52) NYHA II-IV heart failure associated with left ventricular impairment (ejection fraction ≤ 40%). Introduction under specialist supervision is recommended. Contraindications include:
	a. Heart rate < 60
	b. Systolic blood pressure < 100 mmHg
	c. Uncontrolled hypertension
	d. Creatinine > 300 umol/l
	e. Reversible obstructive lung disease
	f. Evidence of fluid overload (raised JVP/oedema)
vi) Spironolactone	For patients with NYHA class III/IV heart failure within the past 6 months and moderate or severe LV impairment on echo. Contraindications:
	a. Unstable angina, primary hepatic failure, active cancer
	b. Creatinine > 220 umol/l
	c. Potassium > 5.0 mmol/l
	(Dose 12.5 – 25mg, check potassium before increment)
vii) Angiotensin II blockers	May be beneficial in patients in whom ACE inhibitors are not tolerated (persistent cough). Avoid in patients already taking a beta blockers and ACE.
viii) Hydralazine and isosorbide.	Consider in those intolerant of ACE inhibitors as a result of renal dysfunction.

Cautions for starting ACE (consider clinic referral prior to commencing ACE)

a) Severe NYHA class IV hart failure and those on >80 mg frusemide
b) Hypovolaemia
c) Patients on additional antihypertensive therapy, e.g consider stopping calcium antagonist prior to commencing ACE
d) History of stroke, transient ischaemic attack or aortic stenosis
e) Serum sodium <130, serum potassium >5.5, creatinine >150μmol/l
f) Systolic BP <100 mm Hg

Figure 9-2. Chronic cardiac failure, part of the treatment description.

ity of the direct patient work. If we can't trust the motives behind a guideline, we're not likely to seek it out and use it, either.

In practice, guidelines are often written to be overly complete, going on for a hundred pages or more, which makes them hard to use in clinical situations. Guidelines written this way are more suitable for concentrated study than for practical application with the patient present, which defeats their primary purpose.

Somewhat unexpectedly, it's hard to find useful guidelines in English, but one decent example can be seen at a site loosely connected to Oxford University (according to the text on the site). The guideline chosen for the purposes of this discussion, is their guideline on the work-up and management of chronic heart failure [12].

This guideline is in the form of a PDF file and summarizes the causes, the diagnostic procedures, and the recommended treatments stratified into levels of seriousness. The guideline document includes text, flowcharts, tables, and forms. Even though the information is solid and useful, the document is a mash-up of different kinds of functionality, all squeezed into one single document, severely impacting its practical usefulness. Let's look at a few aspects of this guideline[3] and its construction, and it'll become clearer just what is meant by that.

In Figure 9-1 we see the beginning of the guideline, where there is a short overview of the basic diagnostic procedures. As doctors we're supposed to know all this by heart, but we don't always remember every detail. It could be too long ago, too detailed, or we can have a bad day, so this is excellent as a brief reminder.

Figure 9-2 shows a part of the therapeutic discussion from the guideline. Again, it's terrific as a reminder, but it is so much more than that. It's also an *up to date* reminder, (or it *should* be[4]), potentially alerting us to changes in recommended therapies caused by new discoveries that may have shown newer agents to be more effective than older agents, or have shown some agents not to be as effective or free of adverse effects as we thought. In other words, however well you know past recommendations by heart, checking through this list can always teach you something new and bring you up to date quickly and easily.

In Figure 9-3 we see more or less the same information, but in tabular form, with indications of trustworthiness in the "Evidence" column, and with literature references in the last column. That last column is essential, since it ties the recommendations to the underlying original data. The guideline should never be an expression of just the author's personal preferences, it must *provably* be based on neutral scientific evidence, and that's where this last column comes in. Without an explicit base in original scientific work, the guideline loses most of its value.

Not everything in a guideline can be based on explicit scientific material, however. Some of it is based on generally agreed good practices, but it's important that those parts of the advice in the guideline are clearly recognized as such. The reader should always have the ultimate say in how much authority she lends to the guideline in the individual patient case, and should not have to take anything in

---

[3] The CHF guideline was reproduced with permission from Dr Chris Bunch and Dr Jeremy Dwight, NHS Oxford, UK.

[4] It's absolutely essential that each guideline includes the date it was last updated, so that we can judge its actuality, but this guideline does not. That is a serious shortcoming.

Chronic Heart Failure

For review and guidelines see: Guidelines for the diagnosis and treatment of chronic heart failure. Task force for the diagnosis and treatment of heart failure, European Society of Cardiology. Eur Heart J 2001;22:1327.

Intervention	Evidence	Summary of results/benefits/risks	Key references
Symptoms and signs and past history	Observational study	The most useful clinical finding in diagnosing heart failure due to left ventricular systolic dysfunction is a displaced apex beat. The likelihood ratio (LR) varies with the presence or absence of other clinical features:	Davie AP, Francis CM, Caruana GR et al. Assessing diagnosis in heart failure: which features are any use? Q J Med 1997;90: 335-9.
		displaced apex beat + gallop rhythm : LR = 44	Badgett RG, Lucey CR, Mulrow CD. Can the clinical examination diagnose left sided heart failure in adults? JAMA 1997; 277: 1712-19.
		displaced apex beat + prior MI + breathlessness : LR = 39	
		displaced apex beat + (crackles or raised JVP) : LR = 24	
ECG	Observational studies	A normal ECG suggests that heart failure is unlikely: among 534 patients aged 17 to 94 patients referred to an open access echocardiography service in Scotland, of 275 with a normal ECG only 6 had impaired left ventricular systolic function.	Davie AP, Francis CM, Love MP et al. Value of the electrocardiogram in identifying heart failure due to left ventricular systolic dysfunction. BMJ 1996; 312: 222.
Echocardiogram	Observational studies	A normal echocardiogram excludes left ventricular systolic dysfunction. In one Scottish study, among 78 patients in primary care taking loop diuretics for treatment of presumed heart failure, 46 had normal left ventricular systolic function.	Wheeldon NM, MacDonald TM, Flucker CJ et al. Echocardiography in chronic heart failure in the community. Q J Med 1993; 86: 17-23.
ACE inhibitors	Randomised controlled trials and systematic review of randomised controlled trials.	Symptomatic heart failure has a poor prognosis eg 4 year survival in the placebo arm of the SOLVD treatment study was 60%. In the same trial the 4 year survival among people with asymptomatic left ventricular impairment was 75%. Among patients with symptomatic reduced LV ejection fractions (heart failure), a systematic review of 32 randomised controlled trials found that treatment with ACE inhibitors reduced all cause mortality by about	The SOLVD Investigators. Effect of enalapril on survival in patients with reduced left ventricular ejection fractions and congestive heart failure. New Engl J Med 1991; 325: 294-302. Garg R, Yusuf S for the Collaborative Group on ACE Inhibitor Trials. Overview of randomised trials of angiotensin-converting enzyme inhibitors on mortality and morbidity in patients with heart failure. JAMA 1995; 273: 1450-6.

Figure 9-3. Summary table with literature references for chronic cardiac failure.

the guideline on faith, or as a result of belief in the authority of the author alone.

When we're working through a guideline, in particular the recommendation parts, we always weight the recommendations against the totality of the patient we have in front of us. Some recommendations can't be followed due to other diseases the patient has, personal preferences of the patient, and many more factors. It's impossible, and unproductive, to even attempt to include all those considerations into a guideline. If we as doctors weren't able to take those considerations into account ourselves, we shouldn't be doing this job, anyway.

But here's a problem. Reading the guideline and selectively applying the advice based on considerations that are not part of the text leaves no trace in the medical record. While the user is reviewing the guideline and reacting to it, she is performing the real essence of her profession, and is taking the important decisions about the patient's care, but it's not persisted anywhere. She can't scribble on the

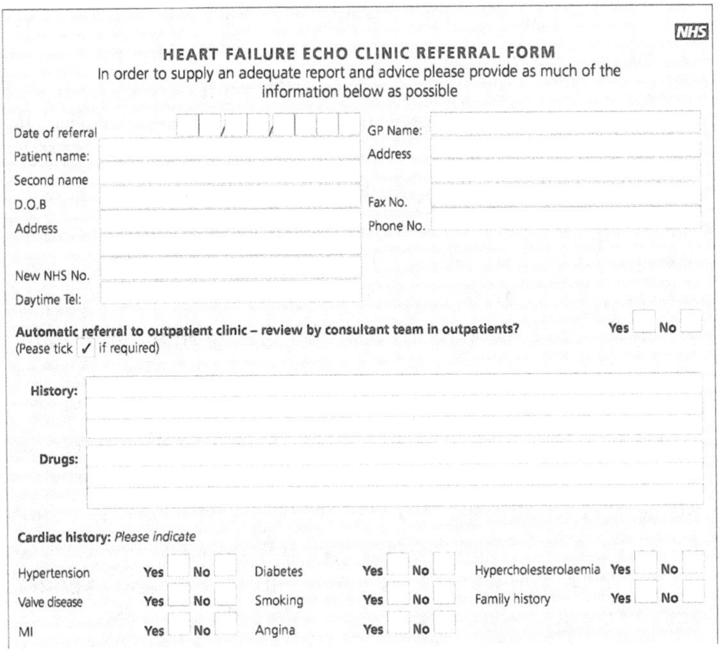

HEART FAILURE ECHO CLINIC REFERRAL FORM

NHS

In order to supply an adequate report and advice please provide as much of the information below as possible

Date of referral / /
GP Name:
Patient name:
Address
Second name
D.O.B
Fax No.
Address
Phone No.
New NHS No.
Daytime Tel:

Automatic referral to outpatient clinic – review by consultant team in outpatients? Yes No
(Pease tick ✓ if required)

History:

Drugs:

Cardiac history: *Please indicate*

Hypertension	Yes	No	Diabetes	Yes	No	Hypercholesterolaemia	Yes	No
Valve disease	Yes	No	Smoking	Yes	No	Family history	Yes	No
MI	Yes	No	Angina	Yes	No			

Figure 9-4. Referral form for chronic cardiac failure.

screen, striking through stuff, or underlining, adding check-marks, etc. The guideline is her worksheet, the very embodiment of her reasoning, and she can't save it? That's ridiculous! In other words, however great the content of the guideline is, the form is wrong. It shouldn't be presented as a read-only web page or even paper document, unless the user can scribble on it, modify it, and make it part of the patient's ongoing record.

The form we see in Figure 9-4 only underlines this fatal flaw. The form is just sitting there, totally passive. Yes, the user can print it out and fill it out by hand[5]. The idea is fine, providing us with the right form, but the delivery is deeply flawed. This form should be different according to the organization and geographical location of the user, be sent automatically to the destination, become part of the patient's re-

[5] Since the death of the typewriter, there's no other way to fill in forms, really. Unless you count spending hours installing and *cursing* Adobe Reader to kingdom come, for the pleasure of *trying* to hit those fields, then *going ballistic* as it can't save the filled in document anywhere, least of all in the medical record.

cord automatically, and become connected to the reply, once it arrives. Clearly, this is too much too ask of a plain dumb PDF file on a website.

In Figure 9-5, we see the final page of the guideline, with a neat flowchart representation of the management of chronic heart failure. This representation is great for a review of the guideline by the user.

There is a somewhat philosophical problem with the flowchart representation, namely that it suggests it could be implemented as a process in medical records, and that would be tragic for two reasons. First, we have the "keyhole" effect discussed in the section "The keyhole effect" on page 121, which results in the user hunting around in the program, answering questions in different ways just to see what conclusions and recommendations can possibly come out of the software. The other reason is that it is an invitation to lay management to try to automate away the need for doctors. The flowchart, after all, seems to indicate that the entire decision process can be reduced to just a few input factors and a few decision branches. Lay people tend not to see what we're using our training and experience for, once the process is reduced to a flowchart. In short, the flowchart here has more potential for damage than for good.

Continuing Professional Education

In most countries, doctors must follow a minimum amount of continuing professional education (CPE) per year[6]. The idea is to bring us up to speed, at least in our own specialty. This idea falls down when scrutinized, though.

The number of diseases we manage as doctors is too large to be comprehensibly covered in any particular year, so a choice must be made as to which subjects are covered. These choices have little relationship to the actual case load of each participating doctor, as a large part of the selection of cases is based on random factors. It's left largely to chance if you will receive training in any one particular subject with any regularity.

Also consider how much you can possibly remember from an education session, and for how long. The information is at the top of your brain, and in a useful state, only for a short time, maybe a couple of weeks at the most. After that, it tends to fade unless it is used

---

[6] Sweden has no such obligation. I don't know what to think of that, really.

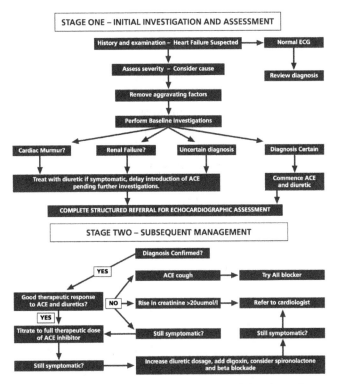

Figure 9-5. Flowcharts for the management of chronic cardiac failure.

and reinforced within that relatively short time period. Any patients with that disease you see while still having the information fresh in your mind will benefit, and possibly make the information lodge more permanently in your memory. But how many, say, Parkinson patients will you see in the first three weeks after that one session on Parkinson you had last year? One?

Others share this pessimism. A paper from the Wellcome Trust [13] says:

> "The researchers estimate that the time lag between research expenditure and eventual health benefits is around 17 years."

That number, 17 years, is pretty much the midpoint of the average career for a doctor, leading us to this informal conclusion:

Nobody learns much of anything after graduating from medical school. Continuing professional education, in practice, makes no useful difference.

Of course, there are exceptions to this very pessimistic rule. Any training in manual dexterity, what is called "craftsmanship" on page 23, is best taught using in-person meet-ups in clinics and operating theaters, or at nice hotels or spas with excellent restaurants and bars, in exotic locations. For theoretical knowledge, however, it is very doubtful that this is an effective method.

CHAPTER 10

How is the record created?

We're entering data into the systems, but how and when do we do that?

Before designing an interface, and even before analyzing the meaning of the entered data, we have to know how and when the user creates the input. It is the physical environment and context around the place and time of input that largely decides the character and value of the data produced.

There are several ways data can be entered into the medical record. There are three major work-flows, each with their own advantages and disadvantages.

Writing afterwards

Some doctors take short handwritten notes during the encounter, then transcribe those into long form notes in the medical-record system after the patient leaves. This implies that the doctor has some time alone between patients, or that she spends time at the end of the day transcribing notes for several patients. If this is done in batch, i.e. for several patients at a time, it becomes harder to not mix up the cases and compromise the information that way.

Usually, referrals, reports, and attestations of different kinds are written in that same period, after the patient leaves. Some doctors write referrals and attestations with the patient present, but leave the dictation or writing of the record for after the patient has left.

Dictating afterwards

In this work-flow, the doctor also takes some brief notes during the encounter, then arranges his thoughts and proceeds to dictate the notes after the patient has left, or possibly after hours. Just as for writing notes in batch, it's easier to mix up the history and findings of different patients if the dictation for several patients is done together like this.

Simultaneous writing

In this work-flow, the doctor takes notes during the actual encounter, as the information is provided and develops.

This way of working is surprisingly easy on doctor and patient. As the doctor reacts visibly by typing to almost everything the patient says, the patient feels he is being taken seriously, is less prone to repetition, and also becomes more succinct and to the point. That's all good.

The major obstacle to this is that the doctor needs to learn touch-typing to be able to maintain eye contact with the patient, at least part of the time. But that isn't hard to achieve with a little training. It's orders of magnitude easier to learn to type well, as compared to learning to become a doctor in the first place.

Another advantage of writing while the patient is present is that if any point is missing or unclear in the narrative, it is much more straightforward to get clarification of these points as the patient is still there to help out.

Finally, since all note taking and writing of referrals is done before the patient leaves, there is no work left to do in the interval between patients or after hours. The patient also gets to be with the doctor for a longer period than if the writing or dictating needs to be done in his absence.

Curiously, in some countries doctors almost always write the record themselves, while in other countries it's rare. It seems to be a cultural phenomenon.

Obstacles to simultaneous writing

The major obstacle is the lack of typing ability in doctors. This can and should be overcome with suitable incentives and training[1].

Another more serious obstacle is the poor design of most EHR systems today. In most of them, it is impossible to refer to all the source documents you need while creating typical output. Often the editor window you use to write notes is the same window you use to look up older notes. The same happens with referrals; while writing a referral you can't go back and read another referral, since these functions utilize the same window.

You can't save a referral as a draft to go look something up, so you need to throw the draft away, go look up something, then start over. Adding insult to injury, you can't reuse an earlier referral, modify it and send it again. Since one of the most frequent work-flows you need to handle is re-composing a referral that was bounced back from a referee[2], these defects combine to form a perfect storm of aggravation.

The systems are much easier to use if you *either* read documents *or* write them, but not both at the same time. It is also often extremely complicated to copy existing information into new forms and notes. Copy and paste is often poorly implemented, and even if it works, it's a very cumbersome method. If you dictate your records, this is not a problem, since the doctor then reads, while the secretary only needs to write while listening to the dictated recording, which explains how this terrible design came into being. The systems are in effect designed for a workaround; having a secretary type the medical record is a workaround for bad designs and defective medical records, and the medical-record system vendors keep designing for that workaround, perpetuating the problem.

---

[1] In Sweden, at least, I'm getting a lot of push-back on this from several reviewers who *can* touch type but are adamant that it's still better not to be distracted by typing while the patient is present. It would be interesting, useful, and entirely feasible, to do an observational study on this, but I'm not holding my breath.

[2] Yes, a "referee" is someone in black and white stripes wielding a whistle, but it also means a person receiving a referral. Look it up.

The way the EHR systems are designed needs to be changed to take simultaneous writing into account. This, again, is probably different according to the culture of the country you're in.

The different results

If the notes are created *after* the actual encounter with the patient, the contents of the notes will be different from those that could have been written *during* the encounter. The reason for this is that in the first case, the notes are an after-construction, where findings are already filtered through the conclusion the doctor reached. It's, in other words, colored by prejudice. As an example, we'll take the following scenario. The doctor listens to a patient telling her about his sore right knee in full detail, and the patient also mentions he had a rash and a fever two weeks before his knee acted up. The rash and the fever will probably not end up in the patient history notes that the doctor writes down, unless she sees a connection between that and the sore knee, the principal complaint. There is no way for another doctor, or a computer, to diagnose any problem with the knee that also involves the rash and fever, by analyzing the notes only. The information needed to do so will simply not be there.

If, on the other hand, the doctor writes down the notes while the patient tells his story, she'll probably write down the part about the rash and the fever long before reaching a conclusion and a diagnosis that does not really involve the fever and rash. As long as the doctor doesn't go to the trouble of going back and erasing that part of the history, thereby intentionally screwing with the veracity of the record, the findings will indeed remain part of the record and may in the future lead to a different conclusion by another doctor or a machine, from the same data.

The greatly increased veracity and usefulness of the medical record in this last scenario, is a strong argument for having the doctor create the record *while* the patient is telling his story, and *during* the clinical examination, not afterwards.

It's of ultimate importance for the objectivity of the data that the record is created as early in the process as possible, during the actual encounter. The only method that can be usefully employed when the patient is present is typing, or dictating, if the quality of the doctor-patient relationship allows it.

CHAPTER 11

The information model

*Current systems are built on a model of the clinical
reality. What does that model look like? Is it correct?*

So, how does the data model[1] look in the EHR, and what can we do
to improve on it?

Legacy EHR systems generally provide a couple of major categories under which they sort the documents belonging to a patient.
These categories are typically:

- Daily notes.

- Referrals and replies to referrals.

- Radiology orders and protocols.

- Lab orders and results.

- Prescriptions.

- General correspondence.

- Forms of all kinds filled in for the patient.

Let's first look at how these legacy systems relate these categories
to each other. Basically, their data model shows the patient as the top,
or root[2], element, and we then have a list of encounters, and another
list of documents. In some cases, the EHR system relates referrals,
prescriptions, notes, and other documents to the encounters where
they were created, but in many systems even this is too much to ask.

---

[1] "Data" is "information" in a form that a computer can process. "Information" is derived from the "data".

[2] In computer science, "trees" have their "roots" at the top. Go figure.

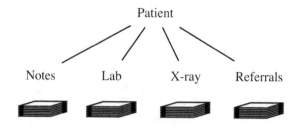

Figure 11-1. The "a few stacks" oriented architecture of legacy EHR systems.

Since the notes from one encounter can relate to more than one problem, while documents such as referrals or prescriptions relate to one particular problem (there are exceptions), the relationship between encounters and documents, if it exists at all, is wrong and misleading. Additionally, documents often arrive outside the context of encounters, such as replies to referrals.

In fact, this organization into separate stacks show a frightening similarity to my Belgian predecessor's stacks I described in "The absence of records" on page 31. We don't seem to have progressed much beyond that, except we now have a significant number of stacks per patient, while there were only two stacks for the entire practice in my Belgian scenario.

For the rest of this discussion, just to keep the diagrams simple, we'll limit ourselves to four stacks per patient, namely: notes, lab, X-ray, and referrals, as in Figure 11-1. The first stack with the notes should really be represented as several stacks if we're talking about large unified systems, since each specialty has its own stack of notes, but still largely share the other stacks (lab, X-rays, referrals, etc) with each other.

The legacy EHR systems have another dimension as well: time. Each of the stacks is organized in reverse time order, so the most recent documents or notes are uppermost (again, just like my Belgian predecessor did it). If we expand the stacks in Figure 11-1 along the time axis, it will look something like Figure 11-2.

In many cases, documents and notes having the same date relate to the same medical problems, but just as often they do not. They may just happen to have the same date for other reasons. In other cases,

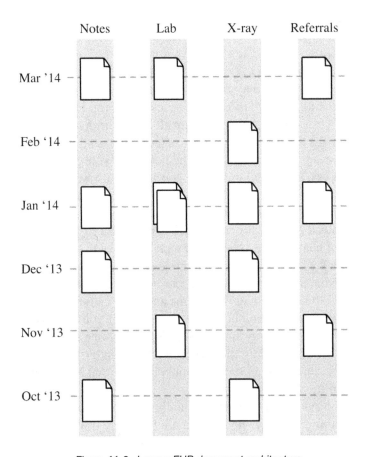

Figure 11-2. Legacy EHR document architecture.

documents that are connected to the same problem or incidence do not have the same date, due to delays in dictation or document creation. This means that the date is a pretty much worthless linking value, and that there is nothing explicitly connecting any particular documents in one stack with related documents in another stack. In other words, if we as users of this system try to gather all the documents and notes that are relevant to a particular medical problem, it quickly degenerates into an error-prone and highly frustrating stack-walking procedure. Let's assume that the patient records in Figure 11-2 contain information on three diseases, one of which is hypertension, which we mentioned in two notes, and for which we've done two lab orders, a chest X-ray, and two referrals (one for funduscopy, the other for a vascular lab). In Figure 11-3 we have marked the documents relating to hypertension with a crosshatched pattern.

The only way to locate the relevant notes is by reading through the stack of notes, top to bottom. After that, the only way to locate other documents that may or may not be mentioned in those notes is by searching through those other stacks from top to bottom. And once you've done that, and have them all neatly arranged inside your head, you just throw it all away again, since there is no way to persist the relationships you just found. The next time you go through the same process, there's no guarantee you'll come up with exactly the same selection of documents from the different stacks, since it all comes down to how attentive you are and how selective, so there is no guaranteed consistency in your view on the record. It's all largely a matter of chance. The more documents there are in the record, the less reliably will you be able to find relevant documents.

Having the documents ordered according to the type of document made sense before we had IT systems and it was all on paper, since that document could only be in one place[3], and if you had to choose between filing that X-ray among other X-rays, or in a folder "hypertension", it made slightly more sense to file it under "X-rays". Not *much* more sense, just a little bit, simply because that X-ray could be relevant to more than one problem.

But with computers, when the number of copies of a document means nothing, it makes no sense at all. An X-ray of the thorax taken during work-up for hypertension has its primary meaning as an exemplar of a study of the *hypertension*, not as yet another X-ray. In other words, the fact that it is an X-ray is just an indication of a method, not of meaning. What we actually were looking for was a possible enlargement of the heart, and to determine if that was present, we used an X-ray. We could just as well have done a cardiac ultrasound, or an ECG, but we happened to do an X-ray.

Now, what happens in the head of the doctor when he reflects on the records and wonders if the patient has a cardiac enlargement? What we would prefer to do is go look in some spot labeled "cardiac enlargement", and find the answer: "no, as shown on thorax X-ray", or maybe "no, as shown on ECG", or even "no, as shown on cardiac ultrasound". But with the stack-oriented EHR systems of

---

[3] Unless we copied it, but that was usually too much work and too expensive.

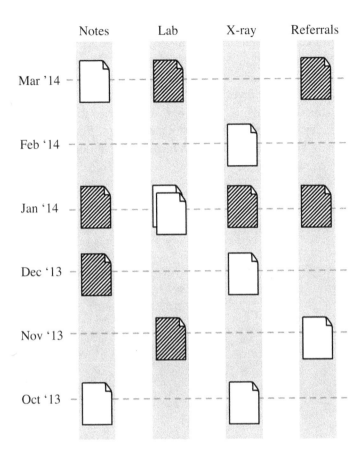

Figure 11-3. Just that one disease is here, here, and here...

today, the doctor instead must assume[4] that the possibility of cardiac enlargement has been verified or excluded using *either* thoracic X-ray, cardiac ultrasound, *or* ECG, and then go searching through each of those three stacks to look for any trace of such an exam[5].

---

[4] That assumption builds on knowledge entirely outside the records, such as conventions in the doctor's area, or that the doctor who did the work-up came from the same university as the reader of the record, or that both the reader and the writer of the record are equally up to date, or out of date, and thus can be expected to use similar methods, etc. There's a lot left to chance, as you can see.

[5] Unless we cave under the pressure and ask the patient, but that defeats the purpose of the medical record, doesn't it?

Even worse, if the doctor didn't know of BNP, a new lab test for cardiac failure, she would not go looking in the stack for lab results after this, and would miss it, if it indeed had been done.

What the doctor *really* wants to know is if cardiac enlargement or heart failure has been verified or excluded, and she really doesn't care much about the method. But what she is *forced* to do with these systems, is try to read the mind of other doctors, figure out which methods could have been used, then backtrack from there.

CHAPTER 12

Conclusion

In this second part of the book, we learned how a typical current EHR system works. We also spent some time looking at how a doctor arranges her working habits around that system, and what the result and pitfalls of these habits are.

Comparing the system and work habits described in Part II with the basic needs of the doctor described in Part I, we must come to the conclusion that there is a disastrous mismatch between the actual need, and what current systems give us. The reason for this is largely found in the chapter on business models and stakeholders.

The mess we are in is caused by having the wrong people define systems for the wrong reasons, and having the systems designed to solve the wrong problems. What a joke.

Part III

A consistent design

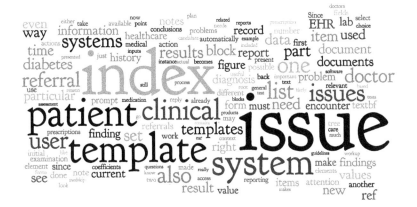

Summary

In the foregoing, we've discussed what the problems in healthcare related to IT are in general, and how current EHR systems attempt, but fail, to solve them. We've seen a number of ways these systems are badly conceived and fail at their task.

In what follows, we'll try to reason out what we need, and how we could go about achieving that. It's clear that we need more than one thing, and that there are a number of aspects of healthcare, that each could use its own solutions.

CHAPTER 13

Necessary, but not sufficient

*Any solution must satisfy this short list of conditions,
else it won't be useful.*

There are a number of specific requirements that need to be fulfilled
for any system to have a chance of becoming useful in practice. We
will briefly discuss each of these core features the system must have.

Effective use

The system must help the user do a better job, do it quicker, and with
less errors. The difference must be clear, and the payback immediate.
The most obvious actions to be taken for a particular issue should be
presented first, and all details that can be taken care of by the system
should be handled automatically.

Finding the right issue, or the right set of issues, to consider,
should be highly automated. Just like an experienced OR nurse who
knows which instrument the surgeon needs next, the system should
serve up the most likely information and tasks before the user needs
to go searching for them. The system should be an assistant to the
user, not just another chore and hindrance.

Context sensitive

The system must be "aware" of the issue at hand. It must adapt and
change its content and mode of presentation according to the set of
issues that the patient has, and which issues are most important at
any particular point in time. The system must therefore filter out everything but the most important, and most likely, actions or inputs.
At the same time, *all* possible actions or inputs should be reachable
in some fashion, of course.

One single system

Legacy EHR systems are a serious millstone around users' necks, and any new system should *replace* it, not add another system to the side of it. The new system should assist the user, *and* produce any documentation that is needed for other purposes. The new system should be the only system the user needs to interact with, and it should form the bridge to any information or functionality it cannot provide itself. There should be one focus, one central management point, one place to find it all, even if some of the content originates in other systems.

Under the user's control

The knowledge-based content (the "issue templates" in our terminology) should *not* be implemented as program code. Instead, this content must be in the form of specifications that any user can create or modify for her own purposes. We can't have a staff of programmers and a development process between any changes in medical practice and the actual implementation of those changes in our tools.

Derivation of issues

The "issue templates" that determine the diagnostic criteria and therapeutic actions in the tool, should be derived from parent templates and allow new templates to be based on older templates. What this means in practice is that any user can take a preexisting issue template, adapt it to her own processes and knowledge, and still keep a connection to the template she derived it from. This allows an easy spread of new knowledge for a certain "issue" to all users of the original or derived template.

   Example: if an institution has derived their own variation of the issue template for "hypertension", their specific issue template should still be updated automatically if a country-wide change of a first choice therapeutic agent is rolled out.

Cover the full process

The system should cover the full process from initial findings, to a
short list of likely issues, and to guidelines for therapy. There should
be full interaction and feedback from each of those stages to the
other stages.

CHAPTER 14

The phases of the clinical process

Observing a doctor working. Fascinating stuff. Or not.

In what follows, we'll discuss the different steps and actions in the clinical process one by one. For each step, we'll first describe the step as such, independent of any IT systems. Then we'll describe how current EHR systems help or hinder this step, and finally we'll go through what future systems could and should do.

Clinical encounter

The encounter can be an ambulatory visit to the doctor, a phone call, or a five minute administrative time set aside to review reports for a patient. It could also be a visit at the patient's bed during rounds. There isn't that much to discuss about the encounter as such, since it mainly consists of a coming together of doctor and patient, at a certain place and time.

How it is

In current systems, the encounter is the main element in the medical record, as far as the notes are concerned. It is reasonably clear what happened and what was examined and discussed during an encounter[1]. At the same time, it's much harder to find out what was done in relation to a particular issue if you don't know when it was done or by whom.

---

[1] "Clear" for arbitrary values of "clarity". What is often not clear are which orders were created or prescriptions written.

The encounter is related to the doctor or nurse, a time, and a place, so if you're mainly interested in that information, it's there. From a medical standpoint, however, this information is practically useless.

Some systems record the creation of referrals and prescriptions right in the notes, but even then, they rarely link directly to the created documents. In other systems, that information isn't in the notes, so it is left to the user to look for documents with the same date and time as relevant notes to try to piece together what really happened[2].

Even if this all works fine, which it doesn't, it helps very little in finding the notes relating to a particular issue, which is really all that matters.

How it should be

The clinical encounters should still be ordered chronologically in future systems, but that is a view that will rarely be used. A better organization is to have notes, documents, results, and prescriptions, ordered according to issue. When the user opens up the records for a particular patient, the very first thing she should see is a list of issues, such as "diabetes", "hypertension", "headaches", and so on. When one of those issues is selected, the user should be presented with a list of plans, notes, documents, results, and prescriptions related to the selected issue.

If, on the other hand, a document, a note, or a prescription is selected, the system should show a list of issues related to that information element, and through that list of issues, the user should again be able to see related information elements, as described in the preceding paragraph.

---

[2] As if that horrible state of affairs were not enough, at least one system I know has a tendency to show the wrong date and time in either or both of those places (notes and documents), making it well nigh impossible to figure out how they relate to each other. That same system, by the way, also records users differently in medication lists and notes, the former with a user login short code, the latter with the full name. In neither place can you see both forms of user identification, so it is *impossible* to match up notes and prescriptions. That reflects some *amazing* dedication to screwing things up.

Overview of the patient history

When the doctor sees the patient, the main things she wants to know about the patient and the encounter are:

- The main problems the patient has or has had over the years.

- Which problem or problems we as doctors need to consider and manage today.

- Which other problems are of importance when considering the current encounter-related problems.

- Which plan is being followed for each of the problems and where those plans are coming from.

- What has been done and decided so far concerning our encounter-related problems.

- What has happened that isn't in the record but is relevant[3]. These are the things the patient should be able to tell us about.

How it is

In current systems, there is nothing but the "history" and the "assessment" fields in the notes to reconstruct the patient's history, unless you count going through all referrals and prescriptions and trying to indirectly deduce from those what could have been the cause of their creation.

History fields are present in each encounter note, so gathering this information implies that you have to scan through all the notes, or all the notes you can stomach, and mentally assemble it all into a consistent whole. If the record system contains notes from a number of different departments, you can choose to go through them separately or all together, if the system gives you that choice. Assuming you're

---

[3] Note that I carefully avoid saying "since the previous encounter", since all too often even important events that have happened *before* the previous encounter are not in the record, and only the patient can inform us of them.

```
2014-01-10        Martin Wehlou, Doctor's notes
Contact           New visit
Reason            Shortness of breath
History           Had similar complaints in 2011, got Salbuterol and improved
                  on that. Last spring also got Pulmicort. Patient still uses
                  both, but is still more affected in cold weather.
                  Pulmicort 200: 1+1 doses per day. Uses Salbuterol every now
                  and then, several times daily.
                  Patient feels pressure over the chest during effort.
Status            BP: 145/85, sitting, left
                  Cor: regular rythm, no souffles
                  Pulm: ves. sounds bilat.
                  ECG in rest: normal.
                  PEF: 225
Assessment        Needs more Pulmicort. I'll order treadmill ECG. Also giving
                  patient an electronic PEF meter for a couple of weeks to
                  collect everyday data.
Referral          Referral sent to UAS, Physiology lab
Prescriptions     Pulmicort Turbohaler 200 micrograms/dose 3x60 doses, renew x2


2014-01-16        Martin Wehlou, Doctor's notes
Contact           Followup
```

Figure 14-1. A typical entry in a classic EHR.

allowed to scan through the notes for other departments without specific authorization and/or reason[4].

During most encounters, we simply skip this step, hoping we didn't miss anything important, but sometimes we simply have to painstakingly assemble a consistent story for some particular purpose, such as a referral or a report to the health insurance. If we do, it's convenient to copy that newly constructed and fairly comprehensive history into the record for later use. The problem, however, is that there is no place to put it except inside the current note, which means that this very useful summary slowly recedes over the visible horizon as later notes accumulate. The only way to keep it current is to keep copying it over to more recent notes, and updating it as you go along, but this is, even at best, a really horrible solution. Some systems have a function to copy old history notes over to the current note, but that's also a really terrible idea, since it results in a large amount of duplicated information, which doesn't get updated any-

---

[4] Since we built up a picture of the patient's history by scanning the notes, it's obvious that we don't really know what we're looking for until we've found it. So we often can't have a known reason beforehand for scanning a particular set of records, even though the reason for doing it would be clear if and when we could see those records. That's some interesting circular reasoning going on here, and the reason for *that* is that the record system is oblivious to the concept of "disease" or problem, so it can't present any information in a cohesive and relevant frame.

way. All you have is then outdated information being added under a current date. You could call it "automated misinformation".

How it should be

There should be a list of issues, aka health problems, over the years, which in itself constitutes most of what we're looking for in a "patient history". The next level down in detail can be found by opening any particular issue and seeing only the notes and documents referring to that one issue. Each issue should contain the *plan* used to diagnose and treat that issue, with a reference to the source of that plan.

For some issues, a time-line can be a good visualization. For example, the long-term parameters and therapy of diabetes have something to gain from a well-designed time-line presentation. Other examples are recurring ear infections in children, or vaccinations, or the follow-up of pregnancies. But there are also a lot of examples of issues where a time-line doesn't make much sense, such as surgery for hemorrhoids or ingrown nails, or a pneumonia. Since the utility of time-lines is so heavily dependent on exactly *which* issue we're talking about, it should be a part of the issue template set for those issues. This has the added beneficial characteristic that the time-line can be designed optimally for each issue type.

There is also the possibility that we'd like to see *all* issues in an overview in the form of a time-line, which could have some utility. In this case, the time-line will be much simpler and not convey much information about each particular issue. Some issues will not be there at all, not in a useful form at least. Just think of congenital diseases like sickle-cell anemia. Yes, each complication of sickle-cell anemia may occur there, but the sickle-cell trait itself can't easily be represented.

For some issues, an anatomical overview could be useful, such as for a multiple trauma, where damaged areas and organs can be highlighted. In rheumatic polyarthritis, an anatomical drawing with each affected joint highlighted can also be very useful.

Clinical examination

The clinical examination consists of a number of manual actions to check on signs and findings. Examples are:

- Listening to heart sounds.

- Listening to lung sounds.

- Palpating the abdomen for masses, tenderness, percussion[5].

- Examining ear drums, eyes, throat, etc.

- Measuring blood pressure.

- Checking reflexes.

Exactly which clinical examinations we do depends on what we're looking for. If the patient presents with an upper respiratory infection, the examination is directed towards respiratory elements. If the patient comes for a yearly checkup of diabetes, we have another set of clinical examinations we ought to perform. Weed and Weed [2] argue convincingly that the initial set of questions and clinical examinations should be exhaustive, so "what we're looking for" should be seen as very broad and inclusionary.

Every doctor knows how to do the most common examinations such as using a stethoscope to listen to heart sounds, palpation of the abdomen, and ear inspection, but other examinations are harder to remember how to do. Examinations for shoulder problems or nervous system diseases can be quite intricate and for these the doctor may need reference material to remind her of which examinations she should do, and exactly how to do them and what they mean.

How it is

In current systems we usually have only a template containing a list of keywords. In some systems you can add keywords or sets of keywords on the fly. If you're seeing a patient with diabetes for a yearly checkup, you would add the set of keywords for just that. But notice

---

[5] Percussion: tapping and listening to the sound. This can tell you the size of the liver, if there's fluid or air in the intestines, and more.

that even if you add that set for diabetes, the system doesn't really take note that you're doing an encounter for diabetes, and doesn't save that fact in any useful way, even though that information is clearly available from the user.

Other systems (or often the same systems, but configured differently) instead have a single or a very few templates with keywords. Since you can't easily add in keywords on the fly, these templates tend to be huge, and tend to include all kinds of keywords that are only rarely used. Often only one in ten keywords are used during an encounter, so much so that the hunting for the right keyword to enter information becomes a significant time-consuming task in its own right.

Both kinds of systems usually only save keywords that do contain entered information into the notes, avoiding saving long lists of empty keywords.

As to how information is entered into the keyword data field, there is very little attention paid to that. Most fields are plain text, with a few fields having a numeric type, which in general is more hindrance than help. Some systems allow for graphing of values over time if the field is numeric, but this has very limited utility since it's done for so few fields. At times it could be useful, such as showing a graph of HbA1c values over time for a diabetic, but this has then to be done by switching over to the lab-results module, then picking out the HbA1c value and graph it from there. It's not a part of the clinical overview for diabetes, simply because no such overview exists.

Another aspect of the use of the IT system in conjunction with the clinical examination is the office layout. A physician's office usually contains a desk with the computer on it, a chair for the patient, and an examining table. These can be arranged such that the computer can be used while at the desk, or easily reached while examining the patient on the table or gurney. But in some setups, the examining room is physically separate from the office, and there is usually no computer in the examining room.

If the examination is done in a room without a computer, the doctor has to either memorize his findings or take notes, the very workflow we try to avoid. If the examination room does have a computer, we're still out of luck, since we usually can't log in to the same EHR system from two places with the same user, either because that was not a part of the design criteria, or because we need a smart card to log in, and it can only be used in one machine at a time.

How it should be

Since the choice of suitable keywords depends on the healthcare issue we're seeing the patient for, it becomes natural to connect the issue to a list of clinical findings. Since national registry, and communicable diseases reporting *also* depend on the healthcare issue, it is obvious that those clinical findings should also be determined by the issue.

Regardless of the reason the user defines the issue, be it in order to get the list of clinical findings right, or to do reporting, or to maintain a correct patient overview, the end result is the same: a descriptive issue in the history overview *and* the right clinical findings for the clinical notes and the reporting.

The "healthcare issue" is such an obvious integrating element that it is hard to conceive how systems continue to be built without that element in their design.

Not only should the set of clinical findings (or "items") be determined by the issue, but the contents the user enters as values into items should be determined by the item. The user should almost always be presented with a default normal entry value, a series of common alternate values, and the option to enter free text. This not only speeds up entry of normal values, but also mildly suggests standard values such that the record becomes more easily exported for reporting purposes, automatic translation to other languages, and coding systems.

The user should never be limited to predetermined choices, only invited to use them. Whenever she bypasses them and enters free text instead, that effort will always be greater than choosing a pre-existing alternative, clearly signaling a defect in the list of available codes. Any such manual workaround of the coding system must be caught and lead to updating of the coding system to fill in the holes.

If the examination room is separate from the office, it has to be provided with a desktop computer mirroring the one in the office. Only one of the machines should be active at any point in time, and the ideal way of achieving this would either be by smart card, which when removed just freezes the screen and keyboard, but does not log out the user entirely. Alternately, a proximity activated system using NFC[6] cards or similar could work.

When designing this, keep in mind that the exam room may be shared by several doctors, so when a doctor activates the desktop, it needs to show the same active session that particular doctor had available moments earlier in her own office.

Another solution entirely could be a portable unit such as a tablet computer, which the doctor can simply carry back and forth and do all of her work on.

Creating referrals and orders

Referrals are created when the doctor wants to have another doctor examine the patient or perform needed therapy. For instance, if we have a patient with headaches, and we can't say with certainty if they're tension headaches or something worse, we may want an X-ray or MRI of the brain, or maybe we want a neurologist to take a look and give an opinion.

In these cases, we start with a problem we can't solve. We have an idea of the general problem area, like "headache" in this example, and what kind of doctor is a specialist in that.

The next step is to find out where there is a neurologist in our geographical or administrative area we can send the patient to. If there are several, we may want to select them according to the patient's preferences or which one has the shortest waiting times.

Once we decide on which neurologist to consult, we write up a referral with the following elements:

- The actual question, such as "headaches of uncertain origin, please advise".

- A short history with major reasons why we can't figure it out, which examinations we've done, and including any results from MRI, lab, etc.

---

[6] Near Field Communication (NFC) cards: those cards you can wave in front of a scanner to get into a building, for instance.

- Related documents in the form of earlier referrals with replies, and documents included with those replies.

After that, we send off the referral using the communication means at our disposal. Sooner or later, the patient will be seen by the neurologist and we'll get a reply back. (See "Receiving results" on page 102.)

How it is

In current systems, referrals, lab orders, X-ray orders, and creation of general documents such as letters and attestations, are completely separate from the notes and from each other. The creation of notes regarding a particular healthcare issue has no influence at all on the document or referral-creating process. Even if the user includes the template keywords for diabetes, nothing in referrals or prescriptions is tuned to diabetes care. Everything is separate and starts from scratch at each use.

If we're having an encounter with a patient for his yearly diabetes follow-up and we open up the prescription module, we're presented with the same choice of thousands of products as always. There is no preselection of products or product classes that are more relevant to our particular patient. The same thing happens with referrals and orders. The range of presented choices is totally independent of the actual problem the patient has, and is therefore always excessive and confusing.

Each document or referral the user needs to produce starts out with a mandatory decision on where to send it. There is no smart preselection of relevant addresses, just a full list of *every* address the system knows of. Also, there is no indication of which addressees are interested or able to handle the problem we wish to present them with, except possibly as indicated by the name of the department. For instance, the "cardiology" department is clearly doing something related to the heart, but do they also take children with heart problems, or do those go to pediatrics? Does the cardiology department do ultrasounds of the heart, or is that the radiology department, or even the clinical physiology department? As users, we're clearly supposed to know all these rules and exceptions, but we don't. This is something the system should do for us.

Next, the user needs to fill in a question (in the case of referrals), and even though we've probably already formulated that in the notes under "assessment" or "planning", there is nothing in the system that makes it easy to reuse that information. Worse, in some systems there isn't even any way of copying that information via the clipboard, necessitating retyping it verbatim.

Finally, we need to rehash the main history of the patient, and the background information we may have. Again, the system won't help us copy over history or assessment notes, or even let us copy over other related documents.

After we send it off, there's a significant risk we'll get the referral back, either because it was sent to the wrong place, or it doesn't carry with it all the information elements the recipient requires. Since these referrals are based on the paper model, the electronic referral now becomes useless, *and has to be written all over again[7]*, even if the change is minimal or only the destination address needs changing. Yes, you read that right; we have to print out the failed referral form, put it down on the table, and proceed to type it in all over again.

How it should be

Since we're working with an issue, the most probable scenarios for referrals should already be provided by the system, with a brief synopsis of which circumstances warrant referrals, and what elements should be included.

Since the issue template is aware of the reasons for referrals, it will also know where to send them, and what should be put into the "cause" field of the referral. It is also aware[8] of the required extra information that the recipient of the referral will need, so it includes that as well from the other sources in the EHR. The only thing left for the user to do is to verify and possibly add a personal touch to the different fields in the referral, then send it off.

---

[7] Accompanied by piercing pig squeals from undersigned, who *still* can't believe how completely moronic the design of these systems can be.

[8] Can't help anthropomorphizing the poor computer. I hope it forgives me.

The chances of the referral being sent at the right time, to the right place, for the right reason, and with the right information, will be hugely increased.

If the recipient, against all odds, still sends the referral back due to misaddressing or insufficient information, the user should be able to update it and send it again, to the same or a different recipient, without starting from scratch. We've had that functionality since forever in plain email, so it's clearly not rocket science.

Creating prescriptions

When we initiate or continue treatments with medications, we need to create prescriptions. When we start a new prescription, we do that with the following considerations:

- The problem or disease we want to treat determines the *therapeutic class* of products we want to use[9].

- We check that there are no *contra-indications* for the use of this therapeutic class for this patient. In other words, does the patient have some other problem that precludes the use of this class of medication?

- We check that the patient isn't already receiving any other medications that may *interact* with this medication. If so, either adjust dosage of one or both medications, or avoid giving one of them.

- We determine the *right dosage and duration* of therapy, depending on the patient's weight, and kidney or liver function[10], and which problem or disease we're treating.

---

[9] To see the whole list of therapeutic classes more formally, see the "Anatomical Therapeutic Chemical" (ATC) classification system [14].

[10] Many pharmacological products are eliminated by the kidneys or broken down by the liver, so if these have a reduced function, the dosage may have to be adjusted accordingly. In some cases, we must do lab tests to determine this, measuring either the liver or kidney function, or the actual concentration of product in blood.

- We locate the information on which *commercial preparations* of this therapeutic class that this particular hospital or region supports or recommends[11].

- Finally, we get around to writing the prescription.

How it is

In current systems, the prescription module is independent of the rest of the system. Yes, it *is* related to the patient and the prescribing doctor or nurse, and department, but not to the current issue, referrals, results from lab, or anything else that is a significant concept in healthcare.

This means that when a doctor sees a patient for a middle ear infection, and she wants to prescribe an antibiotic, the system presents her with *all* the products it is able to prescribe. It is as easy, or as difficult, to prescribe penicillin as it is to prescribe an anti-psychotic medication at this stage. This also means that if the doctor is not certain of the name or type of the product she wants to prescribe, she has the universe of all possible products to plow through, instead of the relatively limited subset of products relevant to ear infections.

In many systems, you can select products according to ATC grouping, limiting the searchable universe somewhat, but simply finding the right ATC group is largely duplicated work. After all, we just told the system what is ailing the patient, so why do we have to keep telling it that in one fashion after another[12]?

Once we've located the product, penicillin V in this case, we need to decide on a dosage. Since the dosage differs according to indication, i.e. the dose is not the same if the penicillin V is prescribed for ear infections, as it is if it's used for pneumonia, and still different from the dose for sinusitis. Even worse, none of these dosages are in the EHR system, anyway. So we have to find the reference information on the product, usually through a web site. Most EHR systems connect to a reference site and do look up the product for us at the

---

[11] Many healthcare organizations make deals with pharmacological companies to get better pricing. These deals result in lists of "recommended products" that doctors are asked (or required) to follow.

[12] Yeah, I do know why. It's because the system is idiotic and doesn't have the concept of "issue" or "disease".

click of a button, but we have to take it from there, scanning the info, deciding on which table of dosages is applicable, switch back to the EHR and enter the dosage in the form. Then switch back and forth a couple of times to make sure we copied it over correctly[13].

How it should be

If we have selected "middle ear infection" as the current issue while examining the patient, the issue template will already contain a list of recommended therapies, including a few different antibiotic classes, so we can choose either the most likely to work, or one the patient is known to tolerate.

When we select one of the products in the issue template, it already comes with a recommended dosage for "middle ear infection", since it's a part of that issue template. The system can easily calculate from there according to age and weight, or ask for the weight if it is needed and not yet available to the system. The duration of therapy is also dependent on the issue, and can be automatically proposed to the user.

In some cases, including middle ear infections, the duration of the therapy can be influenced by prior diseases. If the infection is a first occurrence, the recommendation could be five days of antibiotics, while if it is a recurrence within a few months of a previous middle ear infection, it is recommended to take the antibiotic for 10 days. If the EHR is using "issues", it can easily detect that a similar issue was active less than, say, two months previously, and then suggest a 10 day therapy to the doctor.

We can go even further. For the sake of argument, let's assume the doctor changes her mind about the diagnosis a couple of days later when the therapy doesn't seem to work. For whatever unlikely reason, she wants to change her diagnosis from "middle ear infection" to "hairline fracture of the skull", after discovering that the patient fell down the stairs and having done an X-ray study. She then deletes the issue "middle ear infection" and replaces it with "skull

---

[13] And if our institution is stingy, as large institutions practically always are, we're stuck with a far too small screen with a far too big EHR window, so we can only see *either* the EHR *or* the penicillin V documentation, not both at the same time, hugely increasing cognitive load and risk for errors.

fracture". As she does that, the system can then ask her if she wants to continue the antibiotics, since the system knows that "middle ear infection" is the indication[14] for the antibiotic. It's aware of the *why* of the prescription.

If the doctor removes the issue "middle ear infection", all the data entered into the corresponding template remains available in the EHR, it's only the *framework* of the issue template that is removed. Naturally, both the addition and removal of the template for "middle ear infection" is kept in a history log, but as the diagnosis changes, it doesn't need to remain at the front of the visible record.

Creating the note record

The note record mainly consists of free-form text. One can argue that this is one of both the best and worst aspects of the medical record. It's one of the best aspects since it allows a fully unbounded and expressive description of the patient's condition, wishes, fears, *and* the doctor's assumptions, vague intuitions, and decisions. It's also one of the worst aspects, since it won't allow the computer to anticipate actions, locate suitable support tools, and warn for missing actions and errors.

The note record usually contains the patient history, the clinical examination, and the doctor's conclusions, and open questions, but in this discussion we'll limit ourselves to the "subjective" part[15], the "assessment" and the "planning" parts of the note, since the remaining "objective" part is discussed separately as "Clinical examination" on page 90 and "Finding results" on page 101.

How it is

The "subjective" ("history") and "assessment" parts of the note are currently free text only, which is really all they should be. The problem is mainly that they're mixed in with the clinical examination, results, and planning parts, which they shouldn't be. Taken together,

---

[14] Indication: reason for prescribing.

[15] I'm using the SOAP terms here, but the same applies to equivalent fields in non-SOAP structured records.

this creates a mixed bag of free text, and text that really should be more structured.

In many cases, systems structure a few clinical-examination fields with drop-downs or numerical masks, but this doesn't really make any significant difference, while only being irritating in the cases we need to add something that doesn't fit the preconceived notions the developer had of valid values.

How it should be

We should preserve both the "subjective" and the "assessment" parts of the record as unstructured text. Humans are unparalleled at describing exactly what is perceived, including the degree of un-certainty and vagueness. This description of impressions, state of well-being, and intuitions is very valuable and should not be hin-dered by excessive structuring.

When attempts are made to force the user into using a stricter and more well-defined language in *these* parts of the record, we force the human user to do the work machines are better at, namely syntactic and semantic accuracy, in order to give the machine the task humans are much better at, namely weighting facts and drawing conclusions. In other words, it places both the machines and the humans at their maximum disadvantage[16].

The "subjective" and "assessment" parts of the record must there-fore largely remain textual and unstructured[17]. Since it is hard, or even impossible, to determine exactly which subjective complaints belong to each "issue"—the patient's well-being depends on *all* his problems to some degree—this part should be common to all issues. In other words, whichever "issue" we're focusing on, we should al-ways see the same "subjective" history in full, for that encounter.

The "assessment" part should be shared the same way, since the assessment *must* refer to all the issues the patient has, else it's not a good assessment.

---

[16] For now. In the future, machines will probably do it all. But I'll be dead by then, so that will be your problem.

[17] Colleague Johan M., and others, beg to differ, thinking that even the patient history should be structured. I think that is too much to ask, but time will tell who is right. Or rather, in time Johan will be right, but not for many years to come.

Taken together, this implies that the complete data for an encounter include *one* "subjective" field aka "history", a set of one or more "issues" which contain the clinical examinations, results, planning, etc, and *one* "assessment" field.

Finding results

There are several situations where we need to find replies to referrals, X-ray reports, lab reports, and so on. That could happen during a meeting with the patient, when responding to queries from other doctors, or during planning.

There are three main "angles of attack" when looking for documents, and that is:

- By issue, e.g. everything related to headaches or diabetes. When we try to form an overall picture of the particular issue we're seeing the patient for, this is the most important view. But also, when referring a patient to a specialist for a particular issue, this is also the most fruitful search method.

- By type of document, i.e. X-ray reports, lab reports, replies to referrals, and so on. When considering ordering a test of some kind, it becomes important to see if we have already done that test or examination, or something very similar to it.

- Chronological, that is everything that happened recently, or during a certain time span. This method is more a way of figuring out exactly what was done by us or someone else lately, to see where things are leading. It is often the last choice in searches if the more directed searches don't deliver results.

We refer to results during encounters, since our conclusions are based on these results, among other things. Everything we base our conclusions on, including these results, should be part of the record at that point.

How it is

During the encounter, with or without the patient present, we retrieve a number of results, some of which will be significant for our conclusions and actions. Since it's important to include in the patient record not only *which* conclusions we reach, but *why* we reach them, we have to refer to results somehow. In current systems, there's generally no other way to refer to them except as a textual description. There is then no way for a later reader of the record to with certainty determine what results we used to reach our conclusions, except by painstakingly going through the list of results and matching them up against our, possibly inexact or incomplete, textual description. I haven't seen any system where the textual notes allowed a direct embedded link to another document in the records, but if that could be done, it would certainly help somewhat.

How it should be

If we work in an environment with issue templates, the template itself will have items where it refers to results. If the diagnosis of an infection involves an estimate of CRP[18], the template has the wherewithal to open up the lab reports, then go look for the most recent few CRP values for you. Similarly, if the template contained a possible referral sent during an earlier encounter, it will now go look for a possible answer to that referral and present it in the context of the same issue.

When the doctor then uses the issue template to look up a value and selects the value she chooses to be most significant, that choice is preserved in the issue, making it clear for later readers exactly which result the doctor found most relevant and did use to base her conclusions on.

Receiving results

We also receive results outside the context of a patient encounter. Lab reports and replies to referrals are brought to our attention when they arrive, regardless of what we're really doing at that point in

---

[18] C-Reactive Protein, a blood test that gives an indication of infection and inflammation.

time. Most doctors set aside some time during each day to go through these new results.

When we see a result from the lab, an X-ray report, or a reply to a referral, the first thing we need to do, even before reading the result, is find out why the tests were ordered, or why the referral was written. We need to locate and assimilate the context in which this examination was required, else we won't be able to understand the implications of the results. Ideally, the result should be presented in a reproduced context, with all the notes, other results, and assessments, that were a part of the thinking when the order was created, regardless of whether it was ordered by us or someone else.

If we don't see that context, it becomes uncertain if we will fully appreciate the meaning of the result and there's a chance we will fail to react to it as we would have reacted if we had gotten the result while being in the state of mind we were when we ordered it. If we fail in that way, the result will not be optimally useful, and the care of the patient will suffer.

How it is

Most systems present new results in a list of "new results" or "unsigned results", paralleling the old paper-based work-flow. Back then, we usually got a stack of results dumped on our desks by a secretary, each result attached to the complete medical record of the patient. We were expected to scan the result, do something, then sign off the result in the right lower corner or some other predetermined place on the paper, showing that we did pay attention and from that point on, we would take the blame if the appropriate action wasn't taken.

So here we are in the twenty first century, and we *still* are expected to sign off on the result in a very similar fashion. There's no integrated idea of *why* the test or referral was done, or *what action* we could or should take and if that action did indeed result from it all. The system expects one thing, and one thing only: our signing off on having seen it.

The act of signing off doesn't really imply anything. We could act on the result without signing off, or we can sign off without doing anything else with the result. In some systems, simply *viewing* the result sets a flag indicating it has been seen, while in other systems the user has to click a button (or equivalent) to "sign off", but there is no relationship between this act and any medically significant action resulting from viewing the information.

Worse, the system presents new results in the context of new results, not in the context we had when ordering the test or writing the referral. This leaves it up to the user to go back into the record and figure out when and why the test was ordered and what to do with the result. Far too often, the test was ordered or the referral was created by someone else, under assumptions we don't share, with intentions that were never written down, so we don't know what to do with the result. This is particularly a problem when we're not informed about our predecessor's plan of action, and when *our* plan of action wouldn't have included the ordered test or referral. Due to the lack of context and reasoning, the test or referral result will often turn out to not only waste our time, but also to not result in any useful new plan of action.

How it should be

If a referral is created or a test is ordered from the context of an issue template, that same issue template gets called up and presented together with the result. In this context, the reasoning behind ordering the test is clear and explicit, and the template also contains suggestions on what to do with the result. What the template does is making the plan before, during, and after the test, explicit and clear.

If we're getting the results of a test ordered by a predecessor for reasons we don't agree with, this comes down to not agreeing with the issue template, i.e. the guideline, our predecessor chose, and that is entirely possible and fair. At least we then know our predecessor *did* follow a plan, and which plan that was. With knowledge of the plan and the test results, we have all the material we need to decide on which plan to follow in the future in a fully informed and considered fashion.

Having the originating issue template pop up when viewing a new result also saves huge amounts of time, since all the tools for prescriptions, new referrals, letters to the patient, etc, are right there, for *that* issue. It also saves brain power, reducing cognitive load, and reducing the risk of missing details and making mistakes.

The result should only be taken off the list of "new" results when it has been used for other actions or documents. There is

no point in having a mechanism flag the result as "seen", since having been "seen" means nothing. The user isn't guaranteed, or even likely, to remember having "seen" anything, and even if she did, being remembered isn't something that in itself helps the patient.

We should make a direct connection between removing the item from the "new" list and the appearance of a new note, document, referral, or action in the system. These two events cannot be unlinked from each other.

The list should in fact not be called a list of "new results". It's more usefully referred to as a list of things requiring some kind of action, a "to-do" list. Note well, that even "ignore" is an explicit action for which the user needs to take responsibility. Doing absolutely nothing is *not* an action, so in that case the item remains in the list until some user takes responsibility for creating a note in the record referring to the item, and containing an explanation why it is ignored. That note, in turn, will be assigned to an issue.

If a result or report applies to several different specialties or users, then even if one of the users acts on it, it remains in the unassigned list (the incoming "new" list, if you will) for any other users receiving the same result or report. This way, the result or report will be brought to the attention of all users who need to see it and act on it.

Reporting

Reporting encompasses mandatory reporting of communicable diseases, but also statistical reporting, and case-load related reporting.

To do the reporting right, all the elements needed in the report must be available. These elements often aren't part of the clinical examination and history taking of any particular encounter. To avoid poor reporting or extra work, either all the data must be captured when it's available and used for later reporting, or the reporting should be done during the encounter with the patient[19].

---

[19] Sometimes, the need to report only becomes obvious once results come in, and in that case, it's likely some elements needed for the reporting were not captured, and we have to contact the patient again for that.

How it is

Reports and attestations of all kinds are usually implemented in current EHR systems as a collection of forms with preformatted fields. Some of those fields are filled in automatically, such as patient demographic data, current date and time, doctor's name, and so on. Most other fields are left empty, such as "history", "clinical signs", "conclusions", "recommendations", etc. These fields are often of a character and intention that is dependent on the use of the document.

The same problems referred to while discussing prescriptions (see "Creating prescriptions" on page 96) appear when creating these documents as well. If the user is in the process of handling a particular problem for a patient, only a very small subset of documents is relevant. If the user is treating an infection, reports for communicable diseases may be relevant, but a certificate for a driver's license likely is not. In current EHR systems, the user will still be presented with all relevant *and irrelevant* document forms to choose from, greatly increasing the time and aggravation in finding the right one, while at the same time increasing the risk that she'll choose the wrong form. Which, of course, will come back and bite her later.

Once we get past the onerous work of locating the right form, we have to fill it in. This usually consists of going back and forth a great number of times to look up information in the records, then copying and pasting it into the form, occasionally editing the text to look better, or to fit the form field[20].

How it should be

If the user is working in an issue template for the current problem or disease, any forms that can be relevant for this issue will be listed there, and can be activated from there with a click. This limits the set of possible forms to those that actually make sense for the issue. Nothing hinders the user from going to the full library of forms if she needs something exceptional, but that would rarely be needed.

---

[20] As I'm writing this, I feel my rage boil up again at that one system that for years didn't allow switching back to the record, then didn't allow copy and paste, and *still* even with copy and paste can't handle an excess of text for a form field, simply refusing to paste in that case. Oh, and it won't allow copying less than a full field from the notes either. This is the way you turn plain bad software into an epic fail.

Since the form is linked to the issue, it is easy to link the contents of most form fields to existing items in the issue template, eliminating most of the copy and paste work. Only very few fields will ever need to be entered entirely by hand.

Having the form created from the issue also means that this relationship is preserved. It will be trivial to see in the future that a certain document or report has been created for this issue, and conversely, what issue was the reason for the creation of a particular report.

Reporting to national registries

National registries are maintained for selected diseases or procedures, such as heart failure, diabetes, hip-replacement surgery, and more. These registries can be useful for a number of statistical purposes, and in a selected few cases may even contribute to scientific knowledge[21].

Often reporting is done after the patient encounter by reading the medical record and extracting the reportable data from it. The problem that often occurs is that the right data was not collected during the patient encounter, necessitating contacting the patient again, or submitting incomplete report forms to the registry.

If the reporting can be done in the presence of the patient, or forms (paper or electronic) are provided for the doctor to use during the encounter, the frequency of missing data can be reduced to practically nil.

How it is

In current systems, there is either no help in creating reports to national registries, or forms are provided as lists of keywords in the notes with all the data fields needed for these reports.

Some systems have entry fields in the EHR which clearly make it easier to create complete records with all the required data during the encounter. Better systems also eliminate duplication of entry between the normal clinical examination and the reporting form.

These forms are then checked and completed by a nurse or doctor, then sent to the national registry in binary form (hopefully), and anonymized at arrival. In some systems, the patient identification is

---

[21] I'm sceptical, as you can tell. I'll explain in my next book. Buy it, too.

transformed using some form of hashing function before being sent to the registry. Most of these methods are quite ineffective in protecting the patient's identity.

How it should be

If all required fields for the national registry are part of the clinical issue template, the creation of a report is a simple question of extraction of those data values, and subsequent packaging into a reporting data set.

Before transmission, the data should be fully anonymized and provided with a one-time-only patient identifier, which in turn can only be resolved to the right patient by a designated third party. The technology to achieve this is fairly straightforward, but a precise description is outside the scope of this book.

CHAPTER 15

The real requirements

After removing all the fluff, what's left?

How do we formulate the *real* requirements for an EHR system, that includes the features we need, while not needlessly limiting the solution space? We'll touch on the areas we think are most important.

We'll formulate these requirements as "awareness" key points, underlining the importance of keeping the doctor or nurse informed of the right things, not *how* that information is brought across. It does not matter in the least if it is presented on paper, on a screen, by needle pricks on the back of the hands, or by holographic images in the air. Those are all possible implementations fulfilling these requirements, and it's up to the fantasy and ability of the architects and designers to choose the method.

In the same fashion, input to the EHR system can take any conceivable form, such as typing, speech, gestures, telepathy[1], interpretive dance, or music, but the main point is that it is up to the architects and designers to invent suitable methods. The key requirement is that there *is* an input, not *how* it's done.

Awareness of issues

When seeing the patient, the doctor or nurse must be made aware of all issues the patient has or has had that can have any relevance to the current encounter. The doctor or nurse must also be made aware of the issue that is the subject of the current encounter.

An "issue" consists of a short description of a medical problem or fact that forms the subject for diagnosis or treatment. It should

---

[1] You wish.

be distinct enough to allow identification in the literature, as indication or contra-indication for medication, and as the basis for public-health reporting or statistics. It should be of a form that is, or could be, available in standard coding systems[2] such as ICD-10 or SNOMED CT.

As the user is made aware of the issues, the user should, for each of those issues, be made aware of all the diagnostic and therapeutic steps that have been taken in relation to that issue *and* the reasoning behind it. That "reasoning" includes at least the planning and what scientific basis that planning has, including both diagnostic and therapeutic planning.

Any "summary of care" documents belonging to any issue should also be clearly presented. There should be a way of finding more details than the summary of care presents, but those details could be provided through other means.

Any documents forming the basis for conclusions in summary of care documents, or in responses to referrals, should be included directly or indirectly in these summaries or responses. See Appendix A which is a discussion about referring to sources in the document-tree design, on page 175.

Awareness of patient history

The doctor should quickly and painlessly be made aware of the patient's history in general, i.e. those aspects not tied into a single healthcare issue, but rather related to the whole patient. Things like general well-being, ability to lead a normal life, and the major obstacles to that, including social and financial. This history should not be fragmented and contradictory, but be presented as a consistent whole, where not only the different aspects, but also the evolution over time is clearly shown.

---

[2] If it could be, but isn't, available in standard coding lists, one should take possible mechanisms into account to add the issue to these coding systems.

Awareness of planning

The doctor needs to be made aware of the plans used in diagnosis and treatments, what these plans consist of, the sources they are derived from, and how far along in these plans the diagnosis and treatment have come.

These plans must be explicit and detailed enough so they can be compared with other plans and "current best practice", both by the doctor and the patient. The sources must also be explicit enough so that it can be verified that these plans have not been invalidated by any sources having been retracted or superseded by more recent science.

It should also be clear exactly why these particular plans were selected for this patient: if it was due to the location, the patient's own characteristics, or a preference by patient or doctor.

Awareness of outcomes

It should be clear from the overview what the status of issues is. Are they active, and if so, who is responsible for this issue (doctor, provider, institution)? When was it last managed, and is there any reason to think that it needs more attention? Has it been forgotten about and left without action for too long? Or is the issue resolved, and, if so, how? Or are there outstanding results or responses related to this issue that need handling?

Ensure action

When results or replies to referrals become available, the user should be made aware of these. The system should keep showing these results or replies as "open", or "not yet attended to", until effective action has been taken, and these results have become an integrated part of further decision making. The simple viewing of the result should not be regarded as effective action.

Issue-based management

The patient management should be based on healthcare issues in such a way that the system adapts to the actual problems being managed.

It should be easy to locate a healthcare issue and activate it. Once an issue is activated, the system should present the user with the most frequently used modules and actions that are applicable to that issue. The system should also help the user navigate through the management in the most optimal way, while also helping the user avoid forgetting steps and reminding the user of alternatives, possible other explanations for symptoms, and the expected waiting times and resource costs.

The navigation through a healthcare issue should be defined primarily by the healthcare workers themselves, with the emphasis on correctness and completeness from a medical perspective. The navigation structure and the recommendations are primarily a medical responsibility and form a set of guidelines, but non-medical management can be consulted while setting up these guidelines such that unnecessary delays and costs during diagnosis and treatment can be reduced.

The management of a healthcare issue is defined in what we call issue templates. Such a template contains guidelines for diagnosis and treatments in a checklist form, referral addresses and criteria for referrals, recommended diagnostic means, recommended therapies, and patient information materials.

The system must be designed in such a way that these issue templates can be used nationwide, or be customized for each region, institution, provider, or even patient. There should be a provision for derivation of issue templates from other issue templates, such that the relationship is maintained and it remains clear which templates are local variations of which other templates.

The elements of a template should be multi-lingual in nature, so that the same basic issue template can be used across language borders.

When the management of a healthcare issue is modified due to new knowledge or new resources becoming available, the corresponding issue template should be easy to modify by healthcare workers themselves. At the same time, users employing templates either identical to the changed template, or derived from it, should automatically be given the opportunity to update their own templates, and therefore management, of that healthcare issue.

The issue template is designed to formalize the management of a particular healthcare issue, so it should be made available to the patient, allowing him to judge for himself, or with the aid of another doctor or patient advocate, the contents of the plan, and therefore the quality, of the provided and planned care.

Recording of history

The subjective "history" element is by its nature free text. There is no useful way of structuring this according to some predetermined syntax. Its main function is to report what the patient experiences with as little transformation or interpretation as possible. There's good reason to even let the patient largely write the history part himself.

Since this element reflects the experience of the patient as a whole, it cannot usefully be assigned to any particular subset of issues the patient has, so it belongs to no single issue in the record. It can be a part of any or all issue templates, but the content of the element will always be the same across all issues for any particular encounter[3].

Recording of clinical examinations

Clinical examinations are not in essence different from other items in an issue template. Each clinical item consists of a prompt and optionally a set of preselected values.

While designing the template, we can indicate one of the preselected values as a "default" value, and the system should have a convenient, easy to remember and fast, shortcut or gesture that activates the default choice. Going through a clinical examination, or any other kind of questionnaire that consists entirely of default entries, should be optimized for speed and completeness.

The absolute majority of clinical examination items, even in a very ill patient, will be normal, i.e. correspond to the default value, so the system should optimize for this.

---

[3] This implies that the history part of the record cannot be made available in multiple language versions, unless there's a translation tool provided with the system.

Don't lead me up the garden path

Some legacy EHR systems have warnings for potential errors. The most commonly implemented is the pharmacological interaction warning, which we'll take as an example of everything that is wrong with how these systems are built.

What happens is that you are first presented with a list of *all* medication products you can prescribe, then you're allowed to select one, and only after that will the system come back and tell you it's a bad choice[4]. Now, this just serves to make us hate the system.

What the system *should* do, of course, is only present you with the products that are relevant to the issue you are in the midst of working through. And even *if* it would present pharmacological products that have a contra-indication or interaction warning attached to them for this particular case, that warning should result in a flag that is visible at the point in the issue where you are presented with the opportunity to select a product. In other words, don't waste the user's time by allowing her to select a product the system *already knows* has a warning attached. That warning should be visible *before* selecting the product.

Products that belong to the normal arsenal for the treatment of this issue, but that should not be prescribed due to contra-indications or interactions, should still be presented, albeit with a flag of some kind. If you hide these products, you'll only confuse the user, since the disappearance of a well-known therapeutic product from the issue template could be misinterpreted by the user to mean that the template is defective or the product withdrawn. Also, the interaction or contra-indication warning is just that, a warning, and the user may need to prescribe that product anyway after considering the alternatives and the risks.

The user should always have the ability to choose any product from the total list of existing products, but that choice may reside one or two levels deeper in the interaction hierarchy, since it should rarely be needed if the issue template is well designed.

---

[4] Adding insult to injury: many, if not most, of those warnings are so wrong they're just a waste of time.

Confidentiality

The system must allow for the setting of access limits on issues. This confidentiality flag should limit access in several levels to groups—or roles—of users. The restrictions should not be too detailed, since that makes the system hard to manage. A bare minimum should include the following levels:

- Accessible only to the creating organization (the department handling the problem).

- Accessible to the above, plus designated individual doctors/nurses, or designated other organizations (care centers, departments).

- Accessible to all authenticated medical staff.

Since the access restrictions are set on the issue, not the department, some issues can be confidential, while other issues are not marked as such, even though both kinds can originate in the same department.

The confidentiality setting also includes all medication, all referrals, and lab reports, that originated from the issue in question.

Since the presence of an issue, or any result covered by the confidentiality setting of the issue, can form a warning or contra-indication when another doctor or nurse prescribes medication or orders diagnostic tests or treatments, the system must still be able to warn for that. If the initiating doctor or nurse are excluded from viewing the issue, one of the following actions can be prescribed by policy to occur:

- The originator of the new action will be warned about the contra-indication, and told what it consists of.

- The originator will be warned about the contra-indication, but *not* told what it consists of.

- The creating organization "owning" the hidden issue will be told there is an attempt to prescribe an action that could be dangerous, and this organization will have to resolve the issue somehow.

CHAPTER 16

The full medical process

From illness to cure, every step of the way.

In Figure 16-1, we see the steps that together make up the care of a patient. It's very important to keep the full process in mind when discussing any technology or method that has a bearing on one of these components or steps. Let's work through the diagram now.

Presentation. This is a patient presenting his problem in the most basic form. It could be after an accident, it could be a patient complaining of headaches, or fatigue, or unexpected weight loss.

Initial inputs. The initial inputs consist of the set of questions and clinical signs and symptoms that should be asked all patients of a certain category. All patients presenting a general medical problem such as headaches or fatigue, should be asked the same basic set of questions, and have the same basic set of clinical signs and symptoms checked. If a patient presents a stab wound from a knife, the set of questions will be different, much smaller, and more to the point[1].

Database. The combinatorial database is the set of *answers* to the initial questions, signs and symptoms. (I'm using the term "combinatorial database" in the sense used by Weed and Weed [2].)

Matching. The set of values in the database is now matched against the set of "issues" in the system, to come up with a shortlist of probable and possible explanations for the patient's complaints.

Candidate issues. This is the shortlist of probable and possible issues that could be relevant to the patient.

Additional inputs. The candidate issues, just as all other issues, are each linked to a set of patient-history questions, clinical signs, and findings, some of which are in the set of initial inputs, but some

---

[1] See what I did there?

117

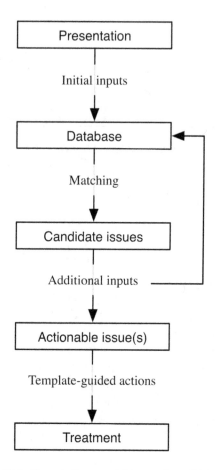

Figure 16-1. Steps in the complete care of a patient.

of which are not. These latter, "new", inputs are now added to the list of inputs, and can be answered by the user and/or patient.

Actionable issue(s). The additional inputs can result in elimination, or at least downgrading, of some candidate issues, and introduction of new candidate issues. The process repeats until there is a stable set of issues which we can act on, which we call "actionable issues". More than one issue can often be the explanation at any particular stage due to imperfections in the methodology. Also, patients may have more than one issue at the same time.

Template-guided actions. Each issue template contains links to the related issue items (complaints, clinical signs, and symptoms), but also the actions that can be taken, such as referrals, orders for X-rays and lab tests, prescriptions, and more. Each of these actions are tailored to the issue itself, so that executing these actions will be much simpler and much less error prone.

Treatment. Once the definite issue or issues have been determined to a satisfactory degree, the actual treatment is chosen from the set of possible treatments available in the issue template (or templates). The choice of exactly which treatments to perform, and exactly how, is something the patient and the doctor do together, where the patient is the primary decision maker. The issue-template advice, however, presents a complete list of options to enable an informed choice, while also allowing a more secure and complete execution of the chosen alternatives.

To make this a living, evolving system, it must be possible to develop each issue template in isolation, and still have the totality of issue templates and input definitions behave as one unified system. Each doctor or institution must be able to contribute their own templates to the system, according to their specialized area of knowledge.

CHAPTER 17

How active should the software be?

Who should run the show? We or the machines?

When the software contains information about diagnostic criteria and at the same time has the clinical data pertaining to the patient, it is tempting to assume that we should let the software draw conclusions from the clinical data and establish diagnoses. Making decisions is what computers are for, after all. But designing for that would be a mistake.

The keyhole effect

If we let the software make diagnostic decisions and pose questions according to past answers, it will lead us through a series of questions and answers that appear to the user in a sequence according to its programming. It proceeds along a path through a flowchart. This hides the overview of the process from the user, giving the user just a "keyhole view" into the exact questions and parameters that the software deems interesting at any particular point of the decision process.

Users will be inclined to game a system like this, simply to be allowed to view the different branches of the decisions tree that are hidden depending on the particular data input. The whole thing quickly degenerates into a charade of false inputs just to make the desired information come up on the screen. Putting in false information into the record for this reason, or for *any* reason, is a really bad idea that is bound to come back and bite you later.

The indiscriminate criteria effect

When the software chooses clinical data to match to criteria, this is often done quite mindlessly, leading to wrong conclusions. For instance, the criteria for the diagnosis of diabetes is, among other things, "two consecutive capillary glycemia values of 7.1 mmol/L or higher".

If we let the software automatically make that diagnosis based on the series of glycemia values in the records, it will make that diagnosis in many cases where a doctor would not, and vice versa. Many of these values may be non-representative, the result of other influences that the doctor knows about, but which the software doesn't. Also, if the software does *not* make the diagnosis, but the doctor does, it will probably force the doctor to falsify clinical data to make the software behave as she wishes it to behave.

If the doctor is made to fiddle with data to make the software draw the right conclusions, the set of clinical data becomes suspect. The right role of the software is to present clinical data and criteria together in an easily digestible format, aiding the doctor as she draws conclusions and makes decisions.

The dis-empowerment effect

If the EHR system is enabled to make decisions that used to be taken by doctors, healthcare providers may see this as a way to reduce the dependence on doctors, thereby increasing the capacity for healthcare, or reducing the costs for doctors, or both. There is nothing wrong with these goals, but there is a significant probability that doctors will see this as dis-empowerment and competition, and refuse to delegate that power to the IT system.

Since getting the cooperation of doctors is crucial to any successful automation project, you should carefully consider if it is worth it to pursue a transition plan that involves taking power away from doctors by force. It is probably more prudent to have that transition occur further in the future, as it will undoubtedly sooner or later be the case, and have that transition be initiated by the doctors themselves.

Nurse vs. doctor domain expert

The leading user influence in EHR development is usually either a nurse or a doctor, and it seems that the difference between the outlook of these two professional groups is severely underestimated.

Nurses usually work in a process-oriented work-flow: start from the top and work your way to the bottom of the list. Typical examples is preparation for operations, postoperative care, post-anesthesia checks, etc.

Doctors seldom work in a directed work-flow, but tend to work with a list of things that should be considered or done, and where the order, or even completeness, is of secondary importance.

A software system designed by nurses will have a fundamentally different work-flow from a system designed by doctors. There is nothing wrong with this, unless you let nurses design systems for doctors or vice versa.

CHAPTER 18

The issue oriented record

It's not all doom and gloom. Issue orientation to the rescue!

In the chapter "Legacy EHR example: Cosmic" on page 49 we saw an example of a current EHR system. You didn't find any description of knowledge support there, because there is none. Nil, nada, zip. We also saw in the chapter "Knowledge support" on page 55 how much we actually need knowledge support in our daily work as doctors. What we *don't* need is another tool to use alongside the medical record, doubling our interactions with the computer. What we *do* need is a tool that *replaces* the medical record as we have it now.

The solution is to take guidelines and other knowledge-based support tools and adapt them so they become both interactive, and a mechanism for recording both history and actions. We'll describe one way of doing just this in what follows.

Diabetes, old style

As an example, we'll use the yearly follow-up of a diabetes patient. There are a number of things the doctor should check, and a number of decisions she has to make. None of these things are very difficult or farfetched, but you have to think of them, and you have to do them.

For instance, you should check the heart and lungs, and take a blood pressure. You should check the weight, the glycemia values, creatinine, lipids, and the albumin/creatinine index in urine. You should also ask the patient how many hypoglycemia episodes he's had the last year. Every three years, you should have an ophthalmologist check the eyes for complications.

The treatment of diabetes type 2 is primarily tablets, and the first choice is currently metformin. If that isn't enough, we can add glimepiride or glipizide.

There's a lot more things like that you have to think about, but the above considerations are enough for our purposes here.

Using a classic EHR system, the doctor has to remember the above items, or look them up in a guideline or book as the patient waits. If the doctor relies on her memory alone, she won't know if the recommendation for, say, metformin as a first choice has changed due to new discoveries. She'll just plow on prescribing it as a first choice forever.

In the classic EHR, the doctor may have a template for diabetes yearly follow-up, with the keywords "Heart", "Lung", "Hypoglycemias per year", "Medications", and "Conclusion", which may remind her of what general areas she should spend some thought on. But that is all. If she wants to make sure the eyes have been checked on time, that's something she'll have to remember to do. And to do that, she'll have to switch over to the referrals module and then wade through it to find any ophthalmology reports about diabetes follow-up[1].

When the doctor orders the lab examinations through the classic EHR, she has to switch over to the lab module, then remember to order the right lab tests for a diabetes follow-up. If she's lucky, there's a preselected group of lab tests for that purpose, but she has to remember to look for that. Back in the notes part of the EHR, there is no automatic indication in the notes that she did in fact order the lab tests at all. That information can only be found in the lab module of the system.

Towards the end of the consultation, the doctor needs to consider any needed therapy changes. She then needs to write a note in

---

[1] There is a dubious assumption here, namely that any examination for eye complications must have been done by an ophthalmologist, and it must have been done due to a referral, so that's where we have to look. What we should have been able to do is find the actual examination results we're looking for, *regardless* of whether it was done through referral, or which specialty performed the examination. The problem is the misguided conflation of *what* was done with *who* did it, that is so pervasive in current systems. The same bad assumption causes confidentiality in current systems to be based on medical departments instead of on the actual healthcare issue.

the record, mentioning if the therapy can remain unchanged, or if it needs updating, and if so, how. If the therapy needs additions or changes, the doctor switches to the prescription module, then edits the prescriptions accordingly. There's no guidance whatsoever from this module about what is the first choice or second choice medications for diabetes. Or anything else, either[2].

We'll stop here, but the rest of the consultation continues in the same vein. Everything medically significant, any real decisions and conclusions, only take place inside the head of the doctor. The EHR system just sits there and allows recording of anything the doctor decides. It assists in sending off prescriptions and finding documents, but it basically has no idea what is going on and why. It has as much to contribute to the consultation process, as a word processor contributes to the jokes in a Terry Pratchett novel.

Diabetes, new style

The new-style EHR tool should adapt to the healthcare issue and the point in time. For each healthcare issue, such as diabetes, it has several variations of templates, each of which is called a "block" in this book. A number of "blocks" together constitute a "template" for a particular "issue" such as for instance diabetes.

For diabetes, there's a block for the diagnosis and work-up, used when the patient initially presents with the problem. There's a block for the yearly follow-ups, which is used multiple times over the years, and there may be a block for the diabetes nurse, and for the foot care specialist, and so on.

The block for diagnosis and work-up is intended to be used once only, and that is when you decide if the patient does indeed have diabetes or not. It also contains the initial examinations and treatments for diabetes. It can be used again if the full work-up couldn't be done in one consultation, though.

Items you'll look at during the work-up are possible infections, dietary habits, weight and weight loss, vascular status, and more.

---

[2] Some EHR systems indicate "preferred" choices, but these "preferred" choices are determined by price, availability, and deals with suppliers, and generally have nothing to do with preference from a medical perspective. As always, the only preferences that seem to matter enough to make it into features, are administrative or financial preferences.

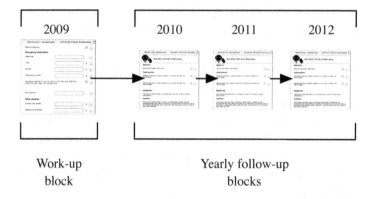

Figure 18-1. The series of issue-template blocks for a diabetes patient.

The actual criteria for making the diagnosis are also evaluated in this phase.

The next type of block is the yearly follow-up block, where we need to go through parameters that indicate how well managed the diabetes is, and if changes of therapy are needed.

After a few years, the patient record will contain several diabetes related blocks, typically one for the work-up, and one for each year of follow-up, and more (see Figure 18-1).

The work-up block

The work-up block, as all other blocks, contains a number of prompts, or questions, that can be answered with plain text, a number, or one of a series of predefined choices. We call each such prompt with its choices an "item".

We should ask the patient about abnormal thirst, excessive urination, sugar urge, infections, and more. We should also check on the patient's general condition, skin turgor (an indication of hydration), sores, Candida infections, or other complications. We need to review lab values for electrolytes, glucose, ketones, and more. If lab results aren't available, we need to order a standard set of lab tests.

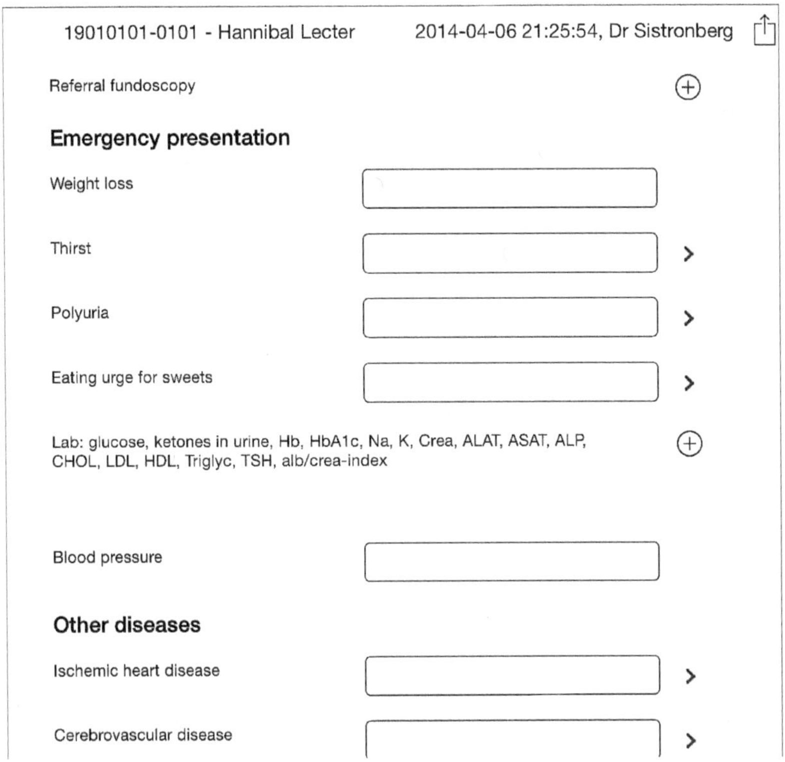

Figure 18-2. Part of the work-up block of the diabetes issue template.

Figure 18-2 shows[3] part of the work-up block for diabetes, where you can see the relevant input fields already provided for weight loss, thirst, polyuria, blood pressure, and more. All these are gentle reminders of what to ask and examine with a diabetes patient at presentation. But you also see the lab tests that should be ordered, and right next to the list there's a ⊕-button to tap which automatically orders just those tests, and then helpfully adds a marker showing they have been ordered. There's no switching back and forth between the EHR system and a guideline system, or between the notes and the lab module in the EHR system.

In Figure 18-3 we see another part of the same work-up block for diabetes. In this part, we're reminded that the diabetes diagnosis de-

---

[3] This and several subsequent images are screen shots from our iotaMed application running on an iPad. iotaMed is an implementation of the ideas presented in this book and does exist for real. Yeah.

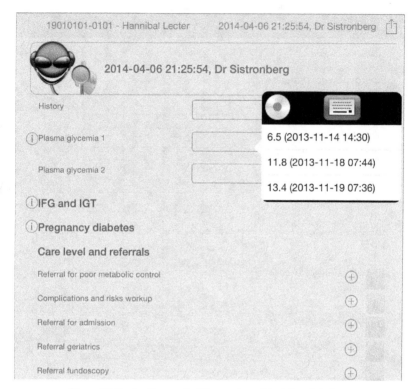

Figure 18-3. Another part of the work-up block for diabetes.

pends on two consecutive values of blood glucose, and by tapping a glycemia field, we get a pop-up allowing us to select the most significant value from the available lab reports. Again, no hunting around different parts of the EHR system to collect the relevant information. Instead, we get it presented exactly at the point we need it, when we need it. By selecting one of the values as most significant, we've also inherently documented that choice, eliminating a bit of note taking at the same time.

If we need a reminder on how high the glycemia value should be for a diagnosis, we can tap (or click, as may be) the info button on the left, and get a brief description of the criteria. Having "information at your fingertips" doesn't get more real than that.

In the lower half of Figure 18-3, you also see a set of useful referrals. Since these are part of the template for diabetes, the referrals are already largely filled in with the right destination, the right questions, and the right included information, as shown in Figure 18-4.

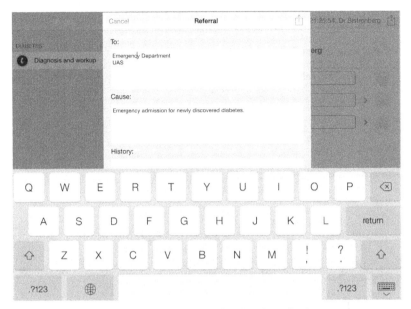

Figure 18-4. Filling in a referral and sending it.

By tapping the ⊕-button to the right in Figure 18-3, the referral form is shown (Figure 18-4), and once sent, it's also marked as completed in the main work-up block as you can see in Figure 18-5.

Therapy

When we get to the part where we prescribe medication, we find the same principles in use. Right there in the issue-template block, we are informed of the first choice medication, with a brief mention of recommended dosages *for this disease* (see Figure 18-6). A number of medications are used for multiple diseases, and for each of those applications, different dosage tables are often used. If the medication recommendation is made part of the guideline in the form of an issue template, that recommendation will be accurate for the issue at hand, without having to force the user to look up the same disease yet again in another system for managing prescriptions.

After the ⊕-button is tapped (Figure 18-6), the system presents the user with a set of alternate recommended doses for this medication, making the selection very simple. See Figure 18-7.

Back in the block, we clearly see the checkmark to the right of the medication, indicating that a prescription was made (Figure 18-8).

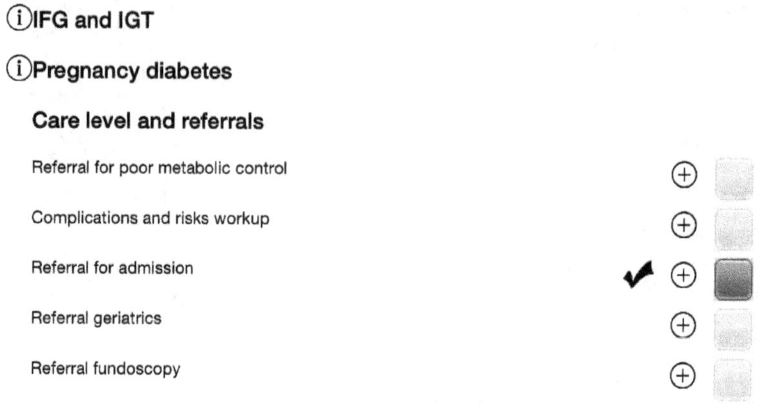

ⓘIFG and IGT

ⓘPregnancy diabetes

Care level and referrals

Referral for poor metabolic control   ⊕

Complications and risks workup   ⊕

Referral for admission   ✔ ⊕ ▇

Referral geriatrics   ⊕

Referral fundoscopy   ⊕

Figure 18-5. After sending a referral, it is flagged in the block.

The square button to the far right is now enabled. Touching that button brings up a history of prescriptions and dosages for that one medication.

With this system, the EHR is "aware" of what disease you are managing, so it can present the relevant medications, and assist in making the right choices. In other words, the most common and recommended courses of action require the least amount of switching around and mental work. The risk for oversight and errors is greatly reduced, as well.

The template structure

With any guideline-based system like iotaMed[4], we have to structure the templates such that they can easily evolve in time as knowledge about the managed diseases improves. We also have to provide for variations in guidelines depending on country, locality, provider, and even at the level of the individual patient. Since an issue template is a digital form of a plan, it must allow adaptation of that plan for any of a large number of reasons.

---

[4] I'm being disingenuous here; there are no other systems like iotaMed.

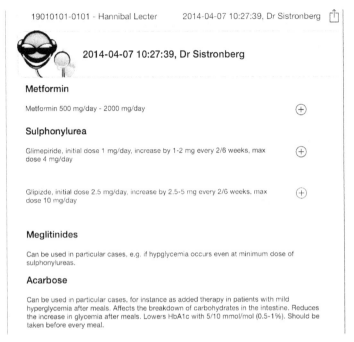

Figure 18-6. The therapy block of the diabetes issue template.

Derivation

The way to allow evolution and local specialization of templates is by classic inheritance and derivation. Any new template is explicitly based on a preceding, similar template, unless you're starting a new template from scratch. The new template contains the identifier of the template[5] it derives from (if any), so that it becomes possible to check for changes higher up the inheritance tree.

To illustrate why this is a good thing, let's assume we have a parent template-block that defines the diagnostics and therapies of diabetes. It contains the defined glycemia limits for making the diagnosis, and the recommended oral medications, among a lot of other things. Let's also assume that a new block is derived for a particular clinic, and that the diagnostic limits are different in this new block, but the therapeutic recommendations remain unchanged. The new

---

[5] Only single inheritance is provided. There's really no need for multiple inheritance in this design. (If that remark went right above your head, don't worry about it.)

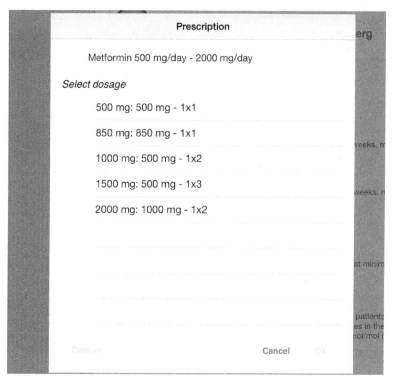

Figure 18-7. Selecting a dose from the recommended set.

diagnostic limits were the reason a derivation was done, instead of using the original template block as is.

At some point in time after this happened, the parent template is derived to a new version with a change in the medication recommendations. Whenever the earlier child template-block is used, the system can now warn the user that there has been a change in medication recommendations in a parent template, and offer to merge in those changes and create a new child template with both modifications together.

The elevator pitch for inheritance is as follows:

By updating issue-template blocks using the inheritance mechanism, any changes to medical-practice recommendations will automatically spread to all users of the system, allowing for an efficient and pervasive knowledge distribution that simply does not exist in legacy EHR systems.

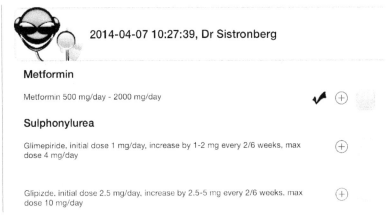

Figure 18-8. Prescription is flagged in the block.

To make this work, all templates and their constituent blocks must be globally indexed, including references to parent blocks and proper security, but the detailed explanation of how this works is outside the scope of this book[6].

Blocks

When we take a regular guideline, such as the one described in "Guidelines" on page 57, and convert it to a template that can be used in an issue-template based EHR system, we quickly notice that the textual information must be subdivided in a particular way to allow it to be useful for a number of patient encounters over time.

For instance, the items in the guideline that concerns making the actual diagnosis are only used and relevant once, at initial presentation, in the form of initial inputs. The items that have to do with yearly follow-ups, however, are revisited at every yearly encounter. This leads us to divide the issue template into "blocks", where each block is applicable to a different type of encounter. In this example, we'd create two blocks, one is the "diagnosis and work-up" block, while the other is the "yearly follow-up" block.

Some issue templates will need blocks for "operation" as in orthopedics, "treatments" as in radiotherapy, "hourly status" as in intensive care units, and even "patient instruction sheets" for helping

---

[6] If you want to know how, hire me.

the patient in his own home care. As an example of available blocks, see Figure 18-9.

Each block consists of a number of elements that we choose to call "issue items", or "items" for short. In Figure 18-10 we see part of the block "diabetes, yearly follow-up". Within the image, there are six "items", each consisting of a "prompt", such as "Foot status", "Peripheral pulses feet", and so on. Next to the prompt is a field for the entry of the value. Some of these fields allow for a pop-up of predefined values.

In the figure, we see that the item with the prompt "Peripheral pulses feet" has its value pop-up open with four predefined values: "Bilaterally present", "Weak left side", "Weak right side", and "Weak bilaterally".

The prompt, the field, and the predefined pop-up values (if present), together form an "item". The item as a whole is defined in a "data dictionary" and can be reused in any number of different blocks, even across issues. This means that if you need to ask the same question about peripheral pulsations in another template block, you don't need to redefine the question and the possible answers, you can simply refer to it from two or more places at the same time. The only thing needed in the block proper is that reference, nothing more.

The actual code that defines the shown part of the yearly follow-up block looks like this:

```
<item name='dd:Hypos'/>
<item name='dd:Status'/>
<item name='dd:FootStatus'/>
<item name='dd:PeripheralPulses'/>
<item name='dd:FootNeurology'/>
<item name='dd:PulmSounds'/>
```

Data definitions

As already described, the items in a template block refer to data descriptions that are defined separately. This allows us to reuse data types in multiple item definitions. So, not only can one item definition be used in several templates, but data definitions can also be used in several item definitions.

The data definition for "peripheral pulses" in the above example looks like this in the data dictionary:

```
<obsdef name='PeripheralPulses' type='select'
                                default='bilok'>
  <prompt lang='en'>Peripheral pulses feet</prompt>
  <prompt lang='sv'>Perifera pulsar</prompt>
  <select value='bilok'>
    <prompt lang='en'>Bilaterally present</prompt>
    <prompt lang='sv'>Bilat närvarande</prompt>
  </select>
  <select value='weakleft'>
    <prompt lang='en'>Weak left side</prompt>
    <prompt lang='sv'>Försvagad vänster</prompt>
  </select>
  <select value='weakright'>
    <prompt lang='en'>Weak right side</prompt>
    <prompt lang='sv'>Försvagad höger</prompt>
  </select>
  <select value='bilatweak'>
    <prompt lang='en'>Weak bilaterally</prompt>
    <prompt lang='sv'>Bilat svag</prompt>
  </select>
</obsdef>
```

All the textual information that can be shown to the user in the form of prompt strings or predefined choices can be defined in any number of different languages. The actual string displayed to the user is taken from the language that closest matches the language of the logged in user. As you can also see in the code snippet, the data definition as such, and each predefined value, also has a "name" or "value" attribute that uniquely identifies it in a user language neutral fashion, allowing automatic translations of at least the predefined values, since what is saved in patient database is the language-neutral value or name only.

If the user enters free-form text, however, that will be saved unchanged in the database, and can only be translated automatically if some other mechanism is used to achieve that.

Both the code for the data definition (the "name" attribute) and the "value" attribute for the predefined values can be replaced or coupled with standard terminology references, such as for example SNOMED CT. This is, as far as I'm aware, the first actually useful application of this term system in medicine[7]. It's unfortunate that the SNOMED CT set of terms appears too incomplete to be reliably

---

[7] Hehe...

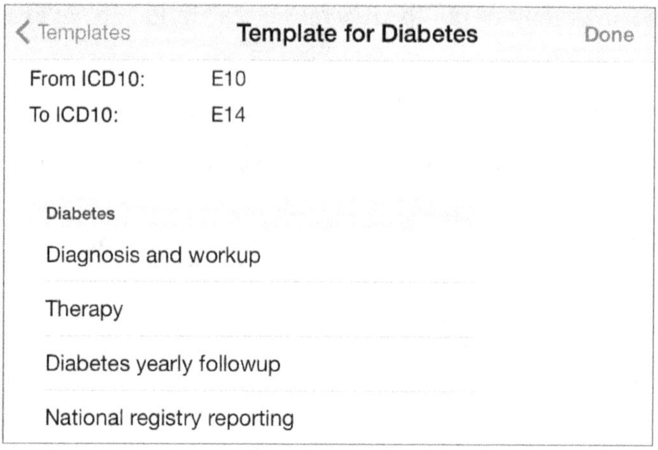

Figure 18-9. The blocks available in the diabetes issue template.

implemented in iotaMed, though[8], which explains why the code examples don't show it.

The data pool

The data pool is the collection of all item data that is entered into all the used issue template blocks for one patient. Each value in the data pool is indexed on a combination of "encounter" and "data definition". The "encounter" is a certain point in time and provider, for instance "Dr Sistronberg" at "Jan 14th, 2014, 15:30".

Since the data value has no relationship to any particular item or template block, *any* reference to one and the same data definition will show the same value for the same encounter. In other words, if you have a patient with a template for diabetes and a template for hypertension open at the same time, you only need to enter a blood-pressure value into one of them to see it in both. This neatly eliminates duplicate work for patients with multiple pathologies.

This separation of data values in the pool from the presentation in a context, as in template blocks, also exactly matches what we in software design describe as the "model" on one hand, and "view" on the other. To put it another way: it doesn't matter if you measure the

---

[8] The Swedish version of the catalogue contains around 400,000 terms, and I *still* can find only about half of what I need for an everyday trivial clinical exam. Amazing, but not in a good way.

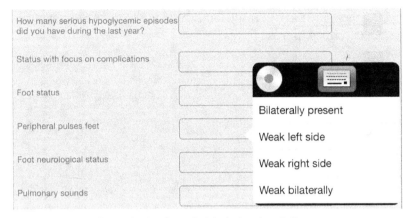

Figure 18-10. Part of a block showing six items.

blood pressure in the context of managing diabetes, or if you measure the blood pressure in the context of managing hypertension, the blood pressure still is one and the same value.

If you have entered the blood pressure into a template block for diabetes, and you then add in another template such as for instance for the issue "cardiac failure" during the same encounter, then the blood pressure will automatically be prefilled into the new template.

When you delete a template block, this does not erase any data values that were already entered. Replacing an erased template block with another does not mean you have to re-enter any values common to both. This allows us to change our mind about diagnoses, deleting and replacing templates, and not to have to repeat already performed clinical examinations.

Checklists on steroids

The issue-template system just described is largely based on the idea of checklists, which have been used in any number of industries and professions for a long time. In medicine, however, the use of checklists is rare and limited, but when they have been used in a systematic manner, they have had a considerable positive impact on the quality of care.

Atul Gawande [15] proposed a brief checklist for use in operating rooms to reduce errors of omission, and these have turned out to be massively beneficial in trials all over the world. Extending the idea by making checklists cover more of the clinical work, and also by making them interactive, results in a system like the issue-template system described in these pages.

CHAPTER 19

Matching findings to templates

Getting from headache to migraine and beyond.

How do we arrange to have the system help us find the right set of templates from a few symptoms? For instance, if the patient has a headache, can't we already present the user with the options "migraine", "hypertension", and "meningitis", just to pick a few?

In the previous chapter, we saw issue templates containing a series of clinical findings, each with a set of alternative values. The template as such works as a checklist, ensuring that the most important aspects of a particular issue are examined and considered by the physician. But these clinical findings have another important function, namely to indicate which *other* issues need considering, leading to a mutual dependency between item values and templates.

For example, if the physician (or the patient) starts out by filling in a very general template, such as one for "fatigue", the values entered should be used to propose other, more specific, templates, such as those for depression, Addison's disease, hypothyroidism, diabetes, etc. Each of those templates should be already filled in with the values entered in preceding templates, and further entry into these more specific templates should lead to further refinement and suggestions for other templates.

The following discussion is heavily influenced by the writings of Lawrence L. Weed and Lincoln Weed in the book "Medicine in Denial" [2]. Weed and Weed describe this matching of clinical findings to issues (or, as they call them, "problems") as the most important advance in medical management we can achieve with computers. It would eliminate the almost random way physicians currently construct diagnostic hypotheses and perform clinical examinations and diagnostic tests. Far too many diagnoses are missed because the physician is incapable of considering the entire gamut of possible routes to a diagnosis, something a computer would have no problem with at all, if it only held the data and the algorithms to do so.

The initial findings

The very first issue template should be fairly simple and it serves to select the major area the problem concerns. This template could consist of a single item (question) with the values (answers) "fever", "fatigue", "abdominal pain", "thoracic pain", "headache", "throat ache", "skin problems", "muscle and joint problems", "trauma", "weight problems", and maybe a few more. Depending on the answer to this first question, more specific issue templates would be activated for further work.

As soon as a clinical finding is entered, the system can present a number of candidate issue templates. For instance, if "fatigue" is selected in the first issue template, the system should already list a large number of possible other issues that involve fatigue, such as hypothyroid disease, diabetes, rheumatic fever, cancer, Addison's disease, and many, many more. Each of these issues have their own set of relevant clinical findings, and a set of these would automatically be added to the active template as the user fills in values.

We shouldn't pick every possible clinical finding from all candidate issues to add to the current template, since that would quickly overwhelm the user. Instead, the most discerning clinical findings should be selected. The selected clinical findings are those that have the highest potential to reduce the number of candidate issues[1].

But that is not enough. We have to have a feedback mechanism such that the system can improve its accuracy as it learns. We also need a mechanism so that "standard problem cases" can be run against the system to verify that the system does not miss these diagnoses.

---

[1] The mechanism used is akin to how an SQL query optimizer selects which index to process first, but instead of having the goal of preserving computing resources, our goal with issue-oriented systems is to as quickly and efficiently as possible reduce the number of candidate diagnoses down to just one or a few.

Combinatorial matching

The term "combinatorial matching" is used extensively in [2] to describe the process of finding diagnoses or treatment from the answers to a large set of questions about symptoms, clinical tests, laboratory tests, and so on. Each combination of signs and symptoms results in a relatively small set of possible diagnoses to work with.

Weed and Weed describe the gathering of signs and symptoms by the physician, or by the patient, with the aid of a computer, as a separate step before the actual combinatorial-matching step, but it

Term	Meaning
Healthcare issue	A disease, or a major symptom such as "fatigue" or "headache", which can have its own clinical findings, and recommendations.
Issue	Short for healthcare issue.
Finding	Short for clinical finding.
Lab finding	The result of a lab test or group of lab tests.
X-ray finding	One or more results from a defined suite of X-ray studies.
Referral finding	One or more results from a referral.
Symptom	Something the patient reports during history taking.
Clinical finding	Any of the above findings or symptoms.
Issue item	The technical implementation allowing the user to enter a clinical finding into an issue block.
Item action	The implementation of the mechanism to create prescriptions, referrals, lab orders, X-ray orders, letters, forms, or other types of documentation.
Issue block	The collection of issue items, and issue actions, and links to background information, related to a particular part or phase in a healthcare issue.
Issue template	The collection of issue blocks for a particular healthcare issue.

Table 19-1. Meaning of terms in this discussion.

could be made more interactive and more effective, if the two steps were merged into one.

We need to define some terms before we proceed, see Table 19-1. These definitions serve the purpose for this discussion, without any claim that these terms are widely accepted. That in itself is not important, but it is important that we agree on the meaning in this context.

Issue items are defined separately from the issue templates and can be used in any number of issue templates. Medically speaking, each issue template contains issue items that either confirm or exclude the diagnosis the issue template defines. If the same item, say "blood pressure", is used in two different issue templates, both templates refer to the exact same issue item definition, *and*, when in use for data capture, the same value. This eliminates multiple entry if two or more issue templates make use of the same clinical finding.

There are three groups of coefficients determining the selection and implications of clinical findings. See Figure 19-1 and Table 19-2. These coefficients together determine which issue templates to consider given how the user has entered clinical findings into items, and simultaneously determine which new items to add to a list of items for consideration by the user. These added items are presented as items in the current issue template view the user is working with.

All these coefficients are determined as part of the process of building the issue template, so they are all under control of the one mind with the most expertise on the subject, with the best shot at achieving "conceptual integrity" [16].

Finding-issue coefficients

When a clinical finding is positive, it will imply that some diagnoses, i.e. issues, are more likely, and some other diagnoses are less likely. For instance, an increase in body weight makes the issue "congestive heart failure"[2] more likely, while at the same time making the issue "hyperthyroidism" less likely.

When the finding is negative, i.e. not present, it will also imply that some diagnoses are less likely. For instance, a normal hemoglo-

---

[2] This is just one of many diagnoses made more likely by increased body weight, of course.

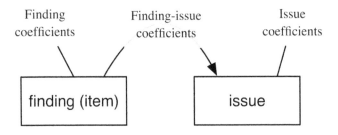

Figure 19-1. The three groups of coefficients relating to clinical findings and issue blocks.

bin will make both polycythemia vera and iron deficiency less likely. A negative finding may, in combination with other findings, increase the likelihood of issues. For instance, if hemoglobin is low (a positive finding), but the average volume of red blood cells is normal, it elevates the likelihood of bone marrow problems[3].

Even though clinical findings interact this way, we don't need to invent some complicated algorithm to calculate these effects. Instead, we'll rely on pattern matching the way Weed and Weed describe [2]. It turns out that the issue "bone marrow problems" has a pattern of "normal cell volume" combined with "low hemoglobin", and therefore is the best match for this combination of clinical findings.

We can construct a set of coefficients reflecting this relationship between the two clinical findings and the three issues as in Table 19-3 and Table 19-4. In the example, we're using the issues "congestive heart failure" (CHF) and an overactive thyroid gland (hyperthyroidism).

As you can see in the tables, values go from −1 through 0, and up to +1. The value −1 indicates that the diagnosis is excluded, and other smaller negative values indicate varying degrees of the clinical finding being an argument against the diagnosis. Positive values indicate arguments *for* the diagnosis in the same way, where +1 would indicate that the diagnosis is a certainty with this positive clinical finding. A value of 0 indicates that the clinical finding gives no indication whatsoever about the diagnosis, either confirmatory or exclusionary.

---

[3] Don't take this text too literally. I'm oversimplifying for the sake of argument, and I really haven't taken all the factors into consideration.

Group	Function of the group
Finding-issue coefficients	This group determines the degree of inclusion or exclusion by a given finding of a particular healthcare issue in the list of likely issues.
Finding coefficients	This group determines how far up the list of questions this particular item (finding) should be placed, other factors being equal.
Issue coefficients	This group determines the sorting of issues that are similarly ranked by other calculations.

Table 19-2. Groups of coefficients.

For instance, from the first table (Table 19-3), we can see that weight gain is an argument for CHF to a medium degree (+0.5), but strongly against hyperthyroidism (–0.9). Fatigue is a good argument for both diagnoses (+0.7 in both cases).

From the second table (Table 19-4), we see that the absence of weight gain says nothing about there being hyperthyroidism or not (0), but is a weak argument against CHF (–0.1). Even if the presence of a finding is an argument for a diagnosis, its absence does not always form an argument against it. It may, but this varies from finding to finding, and from diagnosis to diagnosis.

One can argue that a clinical finding with the value 0 shouldn't even be in the issue template, since it has no relevance to the issue. However, it may be important for pointing to other possible issues, that is, as part of a differential diagnosis. If the user is working through a "congestive heart failure" issue template and answers the question about "tremors" with a "yes", the system could include the "hyperthyroidism" issue template automatically, and thereby also include other fields for clinical findings relevant to the "hyperthyroidism" issue. So a 0 value *does* have a function, albeit indirectly.

If we introduce "general" templates that are used during initial work-up to cover all the symptoms and history elements that should be worked through for every patient, these templates don't correspond to any particular diagnosis, but the finding-issue coefficients attached to these items will result in candidate issues being pulled in and presented as the items progressively become filled in. This is

	CHF	Hyperthyroidism
Weight gain	+0.5	-0.9
Fatigue	+0.7	+0.7
Tremors	0	+0.7

Table 19-3. Positive finding-issue example.

the way we implement the "initial database" that Weed and Weed [2] propose.

The conclusion is that we need to view the influence of findings on the selection of diagnoses (issues) as consisting of two independent parts: the influence of a positive clinical finding on the selection or deselection of candidate issues, and the influence of a negative clinical finding on the selection or deselection of candidate issues. These two influences are generally independent of each other.

Finding coefficients

Each issue item (clinical finding) comes with its own set of coefficients that are independent of any issue templates that may use the item.

The set of issue items to present to the user is determined by the initial general template, and by the selection of candidate issues (which in turn are selected by other items), but the order these issue items are presented to the user is largely determined by the coefficients in Table 19-5. The cheapest, easiest, and quickest clinical questions should indeed be answered first.

Another factor also has an influence on the order of the items, namely the selective ability of the item. The more difference an item can make to the set of candidate issues, the higher it should come

	CHF	Hyperthyroidism
Weight gain	-0.1	0
Fatigue	-0.3	-0.3
Tremors	0	-0.7

Table 19-4. Negative finding-issue example.

Coefficient	Meaning
Cost	An indication of the actual monetary cost of answering the item question.
Delay	Indicates how long it will take to produce an answer.
Discomfort	An indication of pain, discomfort, and general scariness involved in answering the question.
Applicability	A set indicating applicability to genders, races, ages, and so on.

Table 19-5. Finding (item) coefficients.

in the item list. This selectivity is calculated by the system from the finding-issue coefficients described in the preceding section.

Some tests are interdependent or exclusionary. For instance, you should not do contrast imaging of the urinary tract within a couple of days of a barium contrast study of the colon, since the barium will cloud the images. One could imagine any number of expressions or coefficients to take care of all such interdependencies, but that would be overkill. In most cases, it would suffice with a short warning text as part of the template from which you order these test. After all, we're plucking the low hanging fruit here, and we're not trying to automate *everything* away.

Issue coefficients

Each issue template comes with its own set of coefficients, reflecting attributes of the issue itself. See Table 19-6.

The "prevalence" coefficient should not be used to include or exclude issue templates from the list of candidate issues, but can be used to order candidate issues of equal likelihood. If, for instance, a certain set of clinical findings point to both hypothyroidism and sleeping sickness with equal likelihood, hypothyroidism should come first in the list, if we're in Europe, simply because hypothyroidism is more frequent.

The "urgency" coefficient elevates the consideration of certain issues that must be quickly found if present, even if they are not the top contenders in the list of issues. For instance, chest pain usually

Coefficient	Meaning
Prevalence	An indication of how common the issue is.
Urgency	Indicates how urgent it is to diagnose or exclude this issue.
Importance	Indicates how important it is to not miss this issue.

Table 19-6. Issue coefficients.

does not indicate a myocardial infarction, but because it must be detected early if it is happening, it is the first thing we should exclude.

The "importance" coefficient is similar to the "urgency" coefficient, but indicates that the issue definitely should be considered, even if it doesn't have to be immediately.

In summary, we can use the patient's symptoms and complaints to aid the doctor in selecting the correct set of candidate diagnoses. The set of diagnoses conversely informs the system on additional signs to check and symptoms to ask for.

Using coefficients the way that is described in this chapter allows us to let one single system utilize templates created in many different places, by many independent specialists in a scalable manner.

CHAPTER 20

Document tree

*There's logic in how we reason. This is how you per-
sist that logic in the system.*

In an earlier section ("Receiving results" on page 102), we saw how
each received result must include references to all other documents
and other results upon which its conclusions are built. In the document structure we have in current systems (described in the chapter
"The information model" on page 69), this is quite impossible to
achieve. The relationships simply aren't in place.

What we need instead is a document structure in the application
that mirrors how decisions and documents in clinical practice depend on each other. As an example, when we write a referral to a specialist for a patient with some as yet undefined problem of the liver,
we'll probably send along some lab results and the protocol from an
ultrasound examination of the liver. This is shown in diagram form
in Figure 20-1.

In this figure, the top-most element has a double border to desig-
nate that it is a "root", in other words, an element that is not owned or
included by any other element. It's standing on its own, so to speak.
The significance of this will become clear later.

In this example, the specialist performs a liver biopsy and sends
the tissue off for analysis. Somewhat later, the specialist gets a report
from the pathologist about the tissue sample, and uses that tissue
report and the ultrasound protocol that was originally sent to him, to
form an opinion. That opinion, together with the ultrasound protocol
and the tissue report, forms the reply to our referral.

In our original referral, we included the ultrasound protocol and
a lab report. The reply from the specialist includes the pathology report plus the same ultrasound protocol we sent him. In his report, he
refers to the ultrasound and the pathology report, but he never needs

Referral

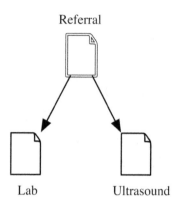

Lab   Ultrasound

Figure 20-1. Referral with two included documents.

to refer to the lab results, so only the ultrasound and the pathology report will be referenced in his reply to us.

His reply will also refer to and include our initial referral request. So what we'll see in the record system after receiving the reply will look like in Figure 20-2. Also note that the reply from the specialist is now a "root" element with a double border. The request we sent to the specialist has lost its "root" double border since it is now referred to by another element, namely the reply.

If the system we're using had a list of "root" elements, that list would initially hold just one entry, the referral in Figure 20-1. Once we get the reply back from the specialist, that entry would disappear, since it's not a root any longer, and would be replaced by an entry for the reply back from the specialist, as in Figure 20-2.

So, what does this mean in clinical terms? Each root is an independent problem, an issue, something we should keep an eye on or react to. After a referral is written, the referral becomes an item to watch, to keep an eye on, until it results in a reply back. As soon as the reply comes in, the referral can be removed (which it automatically is, since it becomes referred to by the reply) and does not need any attention anymore, but the reply itself now becomes an item of interest. That reply *remains* an item of interest, a "root" element, an item in the list, until some other item is created that makes use of it, and it becomes part of a larger, higher-level reasoning.

If we read the reply from the specialist and make a note of that in the records, write a letter to the patient, and create a prescription,

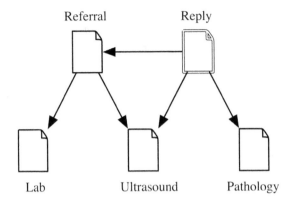

Figure 20-2. The referrer's record data after receiving a reply to the referral.

while referring to all three in our note, we will have replaced the root, that is the element to keep an eye on, with that note. The new relationship will look like in Figure 20-3. In this tree, the note itself becomes an "item of interest". Clinically, this makes sense, since we need to act on it, make it part of something else, classify it as part of a healthcare issue. Maybe that issue could be a "liver problem". When we add that high-level root to the records, it will look like Figure 20-4.

In other cases, the high-level healthcare issue could just as well be diabetes, hypertension, or schizophrenia, for instance. It could also be a symptom which hasn't been clearly assigned to an issue yet, such as "headaches" or "exhaustion". It could also be an incoming request that hasn't been seen and handled yet. The list of current root documents forms a *perfect* overview of the patient's current issues and any elements that are not yet referred to by any other elements. New incoming results will automatically show up in this list and stay there until someone acts on them. As results are acted on, and therefore linked into other actions as sub-documents, they disappear from this list. The only way to remove an element from the list of things "to keep an eye on" is to act on it in a way that makes that element part of a larger whole. The very action on the element removes it from the list. This list fills many of the functions we see in the list of "unsigned" items in current systems, but in a much more sensible and useful way.

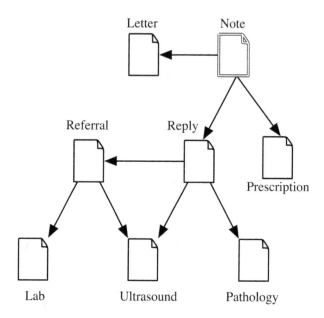

Figure 20-3. The document tree after writing the note.

Another way of looking at the inclusion of documents into other documents, is that they are interdependent. The higher level document *depends* on the lower level documents. If any documents that contain judgment calls or measurement values turn out to be incorrect, then any other documents that depend on them also become suspect. This is inherent in medical reasoning and should be reflected in the document architecture of the EHR system, as it is in this design.

If we start from the top, instead, then we first read the note with our conclusions about the liver problems, and from there we can find and view underlying documents, the one from the specialist, and in turn the pathology report. Clearly, we can reach *all* details that were used in any conclusions this way. Any conclusions that are *not* adequately based on other findings will stand out as a sore thumb.

Interestingly, we can *only* reach the details that have a direct or indirect relationship to the top-level issue we start with, which eliminates a lot of irrelevant information from the context of a particular issue or result. The details that we don't see as part of an issue tree

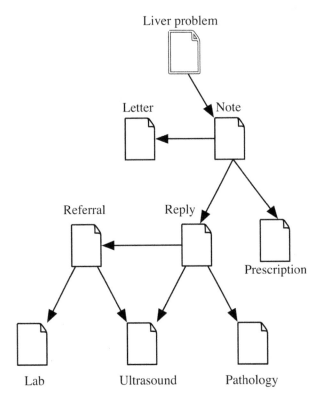

Figure 20-4. After creating the issue "Liver problem" at the top level.

will be shown as part of another issue tree, or if they are entirely free-standing, they will be shown as roots in the attention list.

Elements can have several parents, i.e. be part of several trees at the same time.[1] This is logical, since the same lab result or specialist report can have a bearing on more than one issue. Everything that this shared element depends on will automatically also become shared between both issues.

---

[1] Cyclic graphs are possible, but highly unlikely to occur in practice. As doctors, we don't usually draw conclusions from future events.

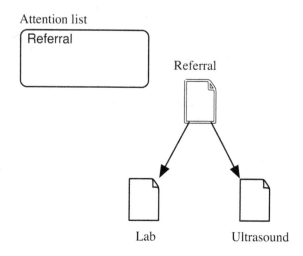

Figure 20-5. Having only written the referral.

The attention list

We've mentioned the "attention list" several times now, but it's necessary to expand on what this means. To do that, let's go through the same example that was used in the preceding section to illustrate how the document tree is built, but this time accompanied by a description on how the "attention list" evolves.

The "attention list" functions as an overview of the patient's issues, while at the same time filling the function of a list of "unsigned items". In fact, it turns out that there is no definable difference between "issues" (or "diseases", or "problems") on the one hand, and "unsigned" incoming results on the other. Both concepts are primary elements of attention and have many similarities from an information conceptual standpoint.

In Figure 20-5 we have just created the referral and included two documents in it, a lab result and an ultrasound report. The referral itself is a top-level element, the root of the tree, and will therefore also appear in the attention list at the top left. When the doctor opens the record, her attention will be drawn to this referral, indicating that it hasn't been replied to, or made part of another attention item in any way. It's freestanding and calling for attention.

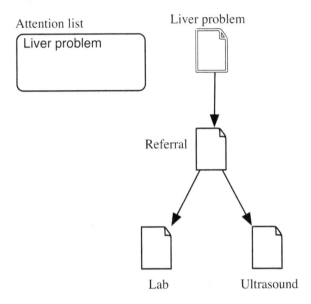

Figure 20-6. The referral has been made part of an issue.

In Figure 20-6 the issue "Liver problem" has been created by the doctor, and the referral she just wrote has been made a part of that issue. Since the root of the tree is now an issue element called "Liver problem", that is the only attention item shown in the list in the upper left.

The specialist receiving the referral, the "referee"[2], gets one document with two sub-documents as shown in Figure 20-7. The referee then creates a reply document which contains links to the referral document, the pathology report, and the ultrasound report that was sent in by the referring doctor. The document set that the referee finalizes and sends back looks like in the Figure 20-8.

When the document is received by the referring doctor, it is linked into her system as shown in Figure 20-9. Both the referral and the ultrasound report were already present in the receiving system, and are not duplicated. The reply is simply linked to those preexisting documents. The pathology report and the reply itself are added to

---

[2] "Referee" is ambiguous, I know. It could mean the patient being referred, or the doctor receiving the referral, but in this text I will use it to mean the latter. I have no other word for that doctor, while the patient can always be called a "patient" instead. So that's what I'll do.

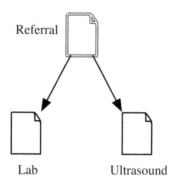

Figure 20-7. The document as received by the referee.

the document tree. Nothing in the existing tree refers to the reply element, so it becomes a second root of the tree (the first one is "Liver problem"), and is added to the attention list. The fact that the reply refers to elements that are already a part of the tree (the referral and the ultrasound report) does not in itself make the reply element part of the tree, allowing us to have it be shown in the attention list.

When the receiving doctor looks at the attention list, she can select the reply from that list, write up a note with her conclusions, base it on the reply, and then write a letter to the patient, and a prescription for a suitable medication. The result will look as in Figure 20-10. The very act of basing her note on the reply to the referral makes the reply a child node and removes it from the attention list automatically. The note itself becomes a new root and will show up in the attention list in Figure 20-10.

The note is in the attention list since it hasn't been yet made a part of a greater whole; it hasn't been properly put into a context. The doctor now selects the note, then links it to the proper issue, in this case the issue "Liver problem", and so makes it a child of the "Liver problem" issue, which automatically removes it from the attention list. The result is an attention list containing a single item, the issue "Liver problem", with no other outstanding items that need attention (see Figure 20-11). Depending on the implementation, this step could be made part of the actual writing of the note in the first place, making the linking to an issue automatic.

One question remains, namely how to view the letter to the patient and the prescription. Is the letter based on the note, or is the note

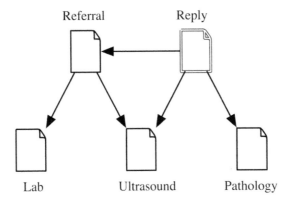

Referral   Reply

Lab   Ultrasound   Pathology

Figure 20-8. The document as returned by the referee.

based on the letter? The same question arises when we think of prescriptions. It is clear that if the letter has no relationships to anything, it should be in the attention list so that the user is prompted to place it into the right context. The same goes for prescriptions. But if there is a link, which should be child and which should be a parent?

It turns out that elements such as letters or prescriptions are a bit peculiar, they're not below or above other elements such as notes, but more to the side of them. Since it would be clinically absurd to put the letter as such as an attention item, or the prescription as an attention item, we will simply make them children of any relationships they are in. They are, after all, results of actions, not causes of actions.

Encryption

We can add an encryption twist to the document tree. Assume that each inclusion of a document at any level consists of a reference to the included document *and* a decryption key so that the referred document can be read[3]. This makes it trivial to read any included documents if you have access to the document that includes them, since that is where the decryption key resides. This also makes it impossible to read a document if you haven't retrieved it by way of

---

[3] For a more detailed explanation of how these keys are handled, please refer to Appendix A, "Document-tree design" on page 175.

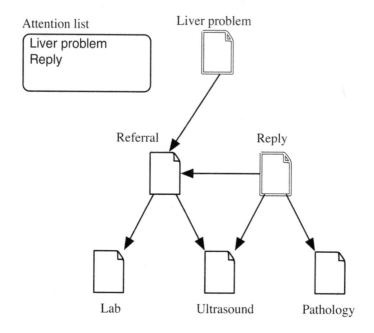

Figure 20-9. The reply has arrived.

another document that includes it. The only way to enter the tree is by way of a top-level document which can be found in the list described in the previous section. From there, you can descend the tree (yes, it's upside down with the root at the top), accessing underlying documents one level at a time.

In fact, this is a very desirable property. If a document has been used as a basis for another document, that base document will always remain accessible to that derived document, but not to any readers who have no access to any document referring to it. In more clinical terms, you can say that if you have access to an issue, such as diabetes, you will automatically have access to everything that is relevant to that issue. In other words, everything that has been considered and influenced decisions about the diabetes care for this patient is available to you. If you have access to another issue, such as schizophrenia, but not diabetes, you will not have access to any documents that are part of the diabetes tree, *unless* those documents are *also* part of the schizophrenia document tree. You will not automatically know that a particular document is also part of a tree you have no access to, but that's how it should be.

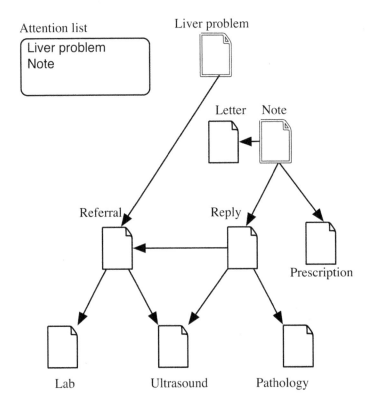

Figure 20-10. The doctor creates a note, a letter, and a prescription.

The document-tree design also neatly implements the abstraction and encapsulation discussed in the chapter "Encapsulation" on page 27. It turns out that this abstraction and division into levels that were described in some depth in that chapter happens continuously with every new referral or response. The document-tree design very closely mirrors how we as doctors think about referrals, which is completely different from how it is implemented in current systems.

In a paper-based medical practice, we would write a referral or response and physically include copies of documents we refer to, such as lab reports and X-ray protocols. If you have access to the referral (by opening the envelope), you implicitly have access to the copies of documents that were included in the same envelope. Since the receiver will base her conclusions in part on those included doc-

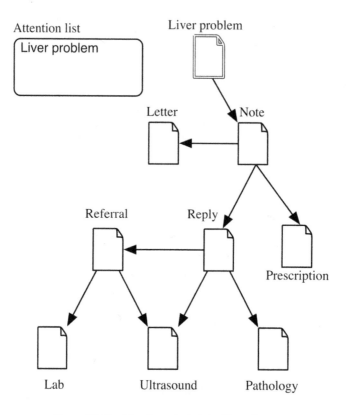

Figure 20-11. After the note is linked to an issue.

uments, she needs permanent access to those documents. In other words, once you've sent them, you shouldn't be able to take them back.

In current computerized medical-record systems with electronic transmission of referrals and responses, this generally turns out to be impossible. There's no provision for attachments in that sense. The solution for the problem seems to be to create huge stovepipe[4] systems, such that the receiver of a referral or result can go dig around for herself in the record system of the sender for those documents that couldn't be attached in the first place. Worse, this seems to be the *major* reason for creating such large unified systems.

---

[4] Stovepipe system: a single huge system doing it all. It's a derogatory term, deservedly so.

In other words, one basic design flaw, the lack of attachments, is incompletely and poorly compensated for by another, even bigger, mistake, the creation of large stovepipe systems.

This poorly conceived arrangement leads to absurdities. In order to give the receiver access to material the sender is referring to, we have to allow the receiver *full access* to a large part of the sender's system. If we ever revoke that access, the access to the referred documents is also revoked, removing any possibility for the receiver of verifying that the conclusions were correctly based on included documentation. The "included" documentation is gone, poof, vanished.

CHAPTER 21

Transitioning and deployment

How do we get from here to there without climbing mountains or upsetting people (too much)?

If we compare the systems of today with the system we ought to arrive at in the future, it's clear that they are quite different. Everything needs to change, including the role and type of work physicians and nurses do. We can't expect this change to be achieved in a single step, nor can we expect the change phase to be limited to a certain period in time. Instead, we must set up a system in such a way that it can be gradually introduced with gradual improvements in processes and outcomes. The system must also inherently lead to further improvements. Instead of climbing a mountain to get to the valley beyond, we need to find a road around the mountain that is always sloping down. Every change we need to introduce must produce immediate payback to all involved parties, or at the very least not introduce any net negatives.

Even though the changes we need to implement are far-reaching and long term, we can usefully describe them in three phases.

Phase 1: guidelines

A large number of guidelines for most common complaints and diseases already exist in one form or another. One particular guideline is discussed in section "Guidelines" on page 57. From that discussion, we can conclude that the content of the guideline is not the problem, as far as applicability is concerned, but the medium and presentation are. It's too hard to locate and use a guideline that is presented in a passive form, even on the web. Also, as already discussed, any use we make of it leaves no footprint in the medical record, making it hard to verify the use after the fact.

Another advantage to starting the transition to a better medical record with the automation of guidelines is that the implemented guidelines will be useful from the start, even if the available number is limited. There is no need to have full coverage of all possible issues to make the use of the tool beneficial. Whatever else is covered by a "general template" as found in most current EHR systems, can be just as easily covered using a general "issue template", with the added and considerable advantage of having the clinical findings and history elements correctly coded from the start. In other words, even if the initial issue template machinery does not have the capability to automatically analyze and suggest differential diagnoses, the data entered in such an early implementation can still be useful in the future, as more advanced analytical tools come on-line.

Replacing old fashioned passive keyword-based templates in current EHR systems with the structured issue templates of an issueoriented medical record makes data entry easier and quicker, while at the same time structuring the data in a way that makes it useful for future tools. It also enables full assistance in the creation of correct referrals and orders.

Having implemented at least a few guidelines as issue templates, already allows for much more efficient and safe prescriptions of medications, creation of referrals, creation of X-ray orders, and lab tests. These features, and the concomitant reduction in mistakes and double entry, will result in huge improvements in efficiency of delivered care, reduction in errors, and higher consistency and quality of care.

These issue-template-based guidelines also provide the ability to warn for contra-indications, *and* they also enable much more useful and accurate management information, by being easily counted and tracked. Each issue template, by its very activation for a particular patient, implies that the issue the template describes can be regarded as "reported" without further intervention by the user.

Phase 2: combinatorial matching

Once there is a significant number of issue templates in use, it makes sense to automatically select matching issues from the set of initial findings. This process would be very similar to the "combinatorial matching" algorithm Weed and Weed describe [2], but the source of the items is not the same as they propose.

Weed and Weed build one single engine that holds all the items needed for an initial work-up, then let that single engine select the issues that match those initial findings. This requires one single code base to be up to date on *all* possible initial findings, and *all* possible issues. In theory this should work, but in practice, it will not scale.

A more maintainable and scalable system would delegate the definition of items, and the definition of issues, to distributed specialists. The execution engine would dynamically build up the set of items to present to the user for the initial work-up after extracting this set from all available issue template definitions. Similarly, the selection of issues from the set of responses to the items should be dependent on the definitions of all included issue templates. This allows the totality of the system to dynamically update itself, depending on all the knowledge inherent in the contributed issue templates.

Phase 3: analysis and feedback

Any computerized decision-making system needs to have a feedback loop built-in, so that the accuracy and precision can be improved continuously and automatically. If a number of physicians use the same system, the system will, as it were, make *all* the users learn from each other's experience and mistakes.

At the same time, the system needs to implement checks and balances, so that the automatic adjustments don't make the system worse or introduce errors, as can easily happen if the feedback system hunts for sub-optimizations to the detriment of global optimizations. This could happen if a particular system very rarely, or never, sees particular issues, and becomes trained not to see that issue at all, causing errors once it actually encounters a patient with that issue.

One way to detect and correct such elimination by optimization is to introduce validation cases, consisting of unusual patient case reports where the ultimate and correct diagnosis is known, to train the system and verify that they aren't missed. A great way of picking up such validation cases is to save those cases that *were* in fact missed by the system. Using these validation cases across a number of systems will make *all* the systems, and thus *all* the users, learn from everybody's experience and mistakes.

Another important element is a review by expert humans of the adjustments made to the parameters in the combinatorial database. This has a twofold function:

1. To detect and correct feedback adjustments gone wrong. Every algorithm has its weaknesses, and an expert human mind can often detect even unforeseen errors this way. Yay for humans!

2. To learn from the adjustments. Each adjustment reflects a mismatch between the expert knowledge of the authors of the guidelines and combinatorial parameters, on the one hand, and the reality of clinical findings in disease, on the other. Some instances of adjustments will be signs of hitherto unknown clinical correlations. Some new syndromes in the form of new groupings of clinical findings can even be flagged entirely automatically by the use of Kohonen maps [17]. The appearance of new groups in such a map could point to a need for new issue templates for that particular group.

Transitioning to an issue oriented system through the three easy[1] steps described above should be possible with immediate gains and payback at each step.

---

[1] Relatively...

CHAPTER 22

Conclusion

Part III of this book started from a clean slate, and took a systematic approach to defining the actual requirements new EHR systems should be built to satisfy.

To do that, we started out by going through the different phases of clinical work, carefully avoiding to define requirements as a function of existing systems, but instead defined them as if no system existed, or as if the system we had was ideal. We took the stance that *all* phases of clinical work should be supported, instead of only the parts that seem important to current, non-medical, stakeholders.

Beyond simply defining the real requirements for a satisfactory medical support system, we also proposed generalized solutions satisfying these requirements, including both a template-based system, and a document-tree architecture, working together to form a holistic solution. The template-based system would solve the majority of the clinical-support needs doctors have when working with actual patients, while the document-tree architecture neatly solves the documentation and retrieval problems of medical records in a way much superior to any current EHR system.

Both these main solution patterns solve the primary problems we have in EHR design, but also, not so coincidentally, solve a raft of secondary problems in information distribution, confidentiality, and auditing.

Part IV

Appendices

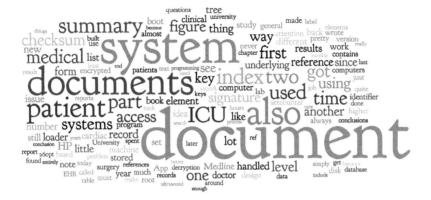

Summary

These appendices are completely optional reading. (As if the entire book weren't completely optional reading, but you know what I mean.)

Document-tree design

*A more detailed look on how medical documents
relate to each other.*

Whenever we as doctors write a summary or a reply to a referral, we always base our conclusions on other documents. It could be lab reports, radiology reports, patient history, clinical examinations, or other replies to referrals. The conclusions we reach are only as valid as those source documents are, with the added ingredient of our own competence and cognition. When we sign off on a conclusion, we do that on the implicit condition that the underlying documents were produced in a similarly considered and reliable way. If any of the underlying documents turn out to be erroneous or ill considered, our conclusion also becomes, at least potentially, invalid. This interdependency needs to be reflected in the way we manage and store documentation. We can't have all the documents in an EHR system just thrown in a heap, but we need to store explicit dependencies of some documents on others.

If we look at a single note in the medical record that contains a conclusion made by a doctor, based on a lab report and an ultrasound protocol, this relationship can be viewed as in Figure A-1. The "conclusion" note itself contains a text where the doctor describes what the lab report and the ultrasound protocol mean, which diagnosis is made, and recommendations for further work-up or treatment. The note with that text also contains links to the mentioned documents, represented as the downwards pointing arrows in the diagram. These links make the dependency of the conclusions in the note explicitly conditional on the content of the two underlying documents (lab and ultrasound).

As each medical specialist in turn refers to a number of base documents, each of these specialists provides a summary at a higher

175

Conclusion

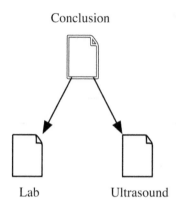

Lab   Ultrasound

Figure A-1. A single note, dependent on two underlying documents.

level than the parts that form the basis for the new summary. The higherlevel summary of the lower-level documents forms the same kind of abstraction that was described in the chapter "Encapsulation" on page 27.

This increasing level of abstraction, which is building on lower levels of abstraction, extends all the way out to the patient, who gets the ultimate summary of earlier and more detailed summaries. In Figure A-2 it is shown that if the patient has access to the root element, the issue itself, he automatically has access to all underlying documents tied to this issue.

If a particular element in the document tree is still on the attention list and not linked to the issue (see section "The attention list" on page 156), and the patient has direct access only to the issue itself ("liver problem" in Figure A-3), he will not see the unhandled element since it is not part of the tree he has access to. If your policy says that patients should only see parts of the record that have been seen and handled by a doctor, this is the perfect technical solution to that.

If, on the other hand, you want to give the patient explicit access to a not yet handled element in the record, you can do so, which automatically also gives the patient access to the underlying documents which that element depends on. See Figure A-4.

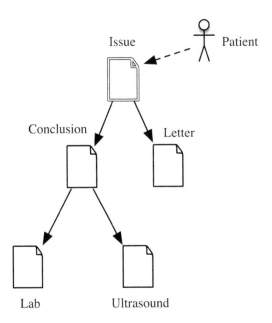

Figure A-2. Patient can have access to the root document, the issue.

Finally, if and when the new note is handled by a doctor and becomes part of the tree rooted in the issue, the patient gets access to that part of the tree as well, entirely automatically. See Figure A-5.

Interestingly, elements at any level which were never part of summaries, or at least not part of any summary the patient or doctor at a higher level ever received, become invisible to this process, which solves another problem, namely how to handle false starts or abandoned hypotheses. Unless these abandoned trails are referred to in any summary that is in the tree we're unraveling, they will become invisible through this process, as they should be[1].

This solves several problems, not least of which is how to hide guesswork and scary little side trails from the patient, if the patient has access to the records. If the scary little side trail had no consequences, it won't become part of a trail of reasoning, and thus not a part of the issue tree, so it won't be seen. It's as simple as that.

---

[1] All elements that have ever been part of the medical record will always be in an audit log, so nothing really ever disappears. Just in case.

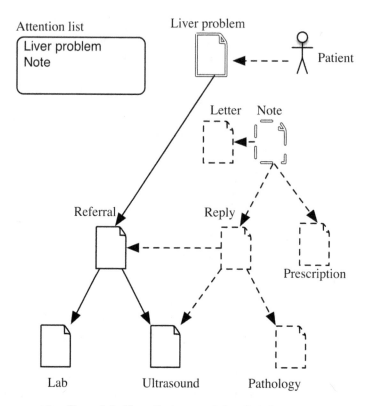

Figure A-3. The patient sees only handled elements.

Interestingly, unused results, notes, replies, and other facts, that do not become part of an existing tree, will form new "root" elements. By visualizing such orphaned roots, we can detect elements that have not been seen, but should have been. Alternatively, these unused and orphaned elements may point to unnecessary use of resources that should be the focus of management attention. For instance, pointless diagnostics which do not contribute to the medical decision process will stick out like a sore thumb.

Another problem we're solving with this pattern is the separation into distinct record systems for different specialties. One way of doing that is hiding all the internal details in a system and only issuing summaries from one specialty to the next. With the document-tree principle, we're in effect doing just that but on a continuous basis, document by document, summary by summary, making the process

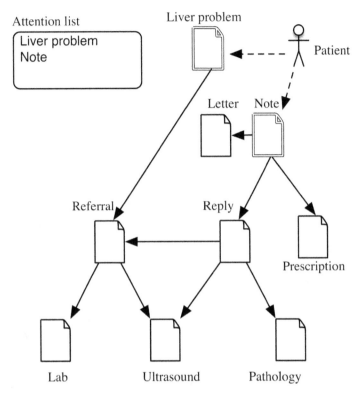

Figure A-4. The patient can be given direct access to unhanded elements.

much more pervasive, and at the same time with no particular border drawn around specialties.

But it gets better still. Since each summary contains not only the references to the underlying documents, but also the symmetric decryption keys[2] for those documents, the underlying documents are fully protected from view from anyone who has no reason to see the document, regardless of where the actual encrypted document is kept. As "reason to see" the document counts being in the possession of another document that refers to it. That document in turn can only be decrypted if the key is retrieved from yet another document higher in the tree referring to it.

---

[2] If you don't know what I mean by "symmetric", don't worry about it. You can enjoy a full and happy life without this knowledge.

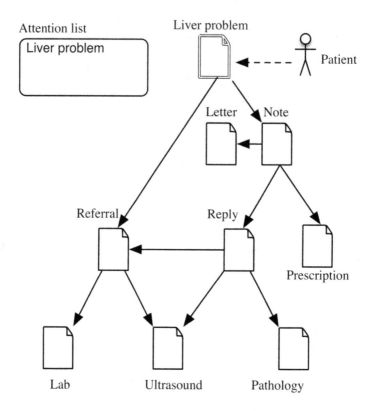

Figure A-5. When the element becomes handled and linked, the patient also gets access.

If a particular document is also used in a scientific study of some sort, it will become part of a collective summary for that study, and thus reachable from the study side. The same documents may, but don't have to, be part of some clinical summaries for other purposes. The meaning and function of "primary data source" used in the performance of clinical studies becomes clear and explicit[3].

It's turtles almost all the way up, but sooner or later you do reach the last turtle, the root, which could be the patient, the GP, or some kind of database, or a clinical-study setup. Each patient could have more than one root, depending on problem areas.

If documents are arranged this way, any constituent documents can have their decryption keys "forgotten" as long as they are part

---

[3] High five!

of a higher level summary. Orphaned document keys could be saved in a special database for useless facts, or simply aged out and discarded[4].

Interestingly, this implies that *all* documents, except the very top level root documents in the tree, can be stored anywhere, even right under the nose of the NSA. As long as the keys to the root documents are safe, the other documents can't be decrypted. Root documents themselves can also be allowed to roam free, as long as the key to each root document is safe. This makes the management of the (momentarily) ultimate keys quite tractable.

The act of "signing off" on received documents, which today is a pretty meaningless hassle, also achieves meaning. As it is in current legacy systems, we look through new results, sometimes signing off on them, but we're never really sure if there is an action presumed on our part, or if the simple viewing of a result has meaning. This confusion is reflected in the implementation of current systems, such that some systems flag results and reports we haven't seen (literally, just like "unread mail" in an email program), while other systems expect us to click a "sign" button, and still others implement both methods in a crazy mix of contradictory messages. If new results instead are viewed as document references that are not made a part of another higher level summary of some kind, then the action expected of the doctor to remove a result or report from the "new" list, is to incorporate that reference in a summary, which could be a note, an outgoing referral, or anything similar. With this system, the actual *action* that makes *actual use* of the result or report, *forms* the signature. There's no ambiguity left. Instead of "unread" versus "read", we have "not handled" versus "handled", or "unused" versus "used", or "uncategorized" versus "categorized", which makes a lot more sense. Every report requires some kind of disposition, else it will stay in the list of the "things that need attention". Neat. (There's a more in depth discussion on these lists of "unused" elements, called "attention lists" in the section "The attention list" on page 156.)

The documents as such, in their encrypted form, can be stored in a distributed-hash-table form or similar, for maximum accessibility and redundancy, with minimal requirements on local database resilience or security.

---

[4] A copy will still have to be kept in the audit log, of course.

Document checksum

What is described here is the technical design to persist these dependencies, while it's up to the designers to make this process transparent and painless to the user. It could be as simple as a clickable symbol inside a document to open any included references to other documents.

First, we need a unique and reproducible reference to documents in general, and the most obvious choice is a checksum on the canonicalized contents of that document. Yes, that was a mouthful, but it can be explained.

A checksum is simply a sum made from the actual text of the document using a pretty complicated arithmetic process.

A "canonical" version of a document is a document where we've normalized spaces and other invisible characters, so that differences between systems should not influence the value of the checksum. We can, for instance, stipulate that all trailing spaces in lines should be removed, and we could specify a particular character encoding in the file, and how the end of lines should be marked[5].

Document signature

A document signature is simply an encrypted form of the document checksum, where the encryption is done using the private key of a public/private key pair belonging to the person signing the document.

The resulting signature can be stored as a pair with the original checksum in a database, allowing us to look up who signed off on a referenced document even without knowing what that document contains. Note that the digital signature contains a reference to the owner of the key, so the identity of the signer can be recovered from the signature as the signature is verified.

---

[5] As an example: Unix-based platforms such as OSX use a single LF character at the end of each line, while Windows and DOS use a pair of characters: CR and LF. Before calculating the checksum we must convert to one of these versions and make sure we always do that, regardless of which machine we're doing the calculation on. If we didn't, a document looking exactly the same to the user would result in two entirely different checksums on OSX and on Windows.

Expression	Meaning
M	The clear-text document.
M_E	The encrypted document.
M_H	Document checksum (hash), which is also its identifier.
M_K	The symmetric key used to encrypt and decrypt the document.
M_S	The digital signature on the document, created by the originator of the document.
M_R	The reference to a document from another document that is dependent on it.

Table A-1. Symbols for document references.

References summary

We can refer to any element from any other by using the document checksum as an identifier. The document can be stored anywhere convenient, and actually locating the document by this identifier can be done in any number of ways, for instance by using distributed hash tables.

The documents should always be stored in an encrypted form, so to access the contents once the document has been located, you also need a decryption key. Each reference to a document must therefore include two elements: the document reference (which is equal to its checksum), and the decryption key. These are described using the symbols defined in Table A-1. The letter "*M*" denotes "message" in crypto lingo, but in this case the "message" is the same thing as "document" or "element of the record".

With this notation, we see that a reference to a document must include two things: the document identifier (so we can locate it), and the symmetric encryption key (so we can read it):

$$M_R = \{M_H, M_K\}$$

The document itself, in its encrypted form, is stored together with its identifier, so it can be located:

$$\{M_H, M_E\}$$

The document signature can be kept separately. It also needs the document identifier so we can find it and link it to the document it signs:

$$\{M_H, M_S\}$$

Since the checksum was calculated on the plain text form of the document, it cannot be verified to be correct until after the decryption of the document. The same limitation applies to the digital signature; the document must be decrypted before it can be verified.

Unique reference problem

There is a potential for document reference collisions with the system as described. If the exact same document is encrypted and stored from two different locations, we could have two stored documents with the same reference and different encryption keys. If we mandate document reference uniqueness, either the later document will overwrite the earlier, or the later document cannot be stored at all.

One way of avoiding this situation is to never allow documents to be distributed in clear text, which implies that every document is immediatly encrypted and stored on creation, as they should be. The only distribution mechanism is then by reference to the encrypted and stored form.

Another, less desirable, solution is to slightly modify the later stored documents such that they result in a different checksum, and basically become different documents. We may have to do this when importing legacy medical documentation into a document tree.

Other solutions of variable suitability exist, but discussing those in these pages would take us far away on numerous tangents. Let's just keep in mind that this problem exists and will be most prominent during a transition period.

About the author

What happened to me, to make this book happen to you?

There's no avoiding a section on who I am. This book is based almost entirely on my own experiences, and this both liberates me and forms a limitation on the applicability of my conclusions. There must be a large number of situations where my descriptions are invalid, but there is very little other literature to base any comparison on. I'll simply have to describe my experiences and let you draw your own conclusions as to why I'm saying what I'm saying. I'll include a lot of details, but I'll try to be brief, since this isn't supposed to be a biography, but a book about the EHR.

I was born and grew up in Stockholm, Sweden, attending Stockholm University between 1969 and 1971, studying mathematics, a sprinkling of programming (ALGOL, if anyone remembers that), and inorganic chemistry.

In 1971 I moved to Ghent, Belgium, studying medicine at the state university between 1971 and 1978, graduated with honors. During my last year of internship, I once got the task of reprogramming a small part of an analysis automation package for clinical chemistry on a PDP-8 running Focal.

Between 1978 and 1983, I did a general surgery residency at the same university. This included six months of orthopedics and quite a bit of intensive care. Vascular and thoracic surgery was also part of the daily work. The training didn't include cardiac surgery as such, but each resident assisted hundreds of coronary bypass and valve replacement procedures, and a smaller number of pediatric cardiac operations.

During this residency, I stumbled across an HP 2100A mini computer in a back room of the ICU. This machine had an A/D converter,

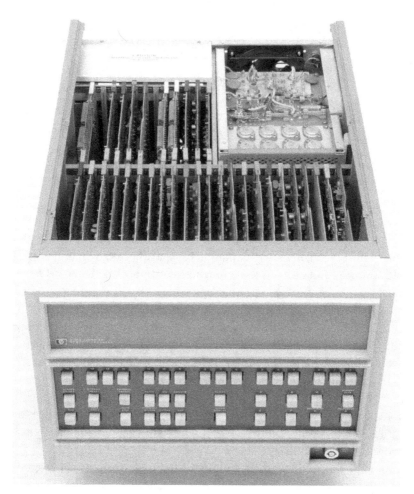

Figure B-1. The main unit of the HP 2100A mini computer. (Photo courtesy of hpmemory.org, Marc Mislanghe.)

a *huge* 14 inch removable disk and a fixed hard disk of the same size, each almost 2.4 megabytes in capacity. The RAM was 32k words (64k bytes), and the clock frequency around 1 MHz. I found terminals and other peripherals in the basement and other departments, and hooked them up. I ended up with a teletype console, a Tektronix vector graphic terminal, an HP block-mode terminal, a few cheaper terminals I've forgotten the name of, and a couple of little 8" (or so) graphic displays with 256 x 256 pixels[1].

---

[1] I may mis-remember details, could be less, or it could be more.

The A/D converter had 128 channels and was still hooked up to a number of bedside monitors in the ICU. It used DMA and kernel processes to write directly to disk and could read at 50 samples per second.

The entire system was housed in two 19 inch racks bolted to the floor. When the hard disk got going really well, it would have tipped over the racks otherwise.

The way to boot this monster was interesting. Assuming it lost all track of reality, the first thing you had to do was insert a physical key and unlock the last 32 words in memory, so you could punch in the first bootstrap loader, the "loader loader", using front panel illuminated buttons, all in binary. (After about a hundred times, I knew this boot-loader-loader binary by heart.) After entering the boot-loader-loader binary, you removed the key, locking down the memory[2], set the instruction counter to the start of the boot-loader loader, inserted the disk-operating-system boot-loader paper tape in the paper-tape reader, then hit "run". The paper tape ran through the reader at an amazing speed, hitting the wall almost two meters to the left. Then the disk boot got going, the RTE-III "Real Time Executive" was loaded, and after a while you got the satisfying hum and clunk from the teletype.

Residents had to stay over in the hospital two or three nights a week, while not getting any days off, so we spent 80 or 90 hours a week at work. We slept some, of course, but never enough. Once I found this HP 2100, I hardly ever slept, instead spending my nights figuring out how to reconfigure it using "system generations", and how to program it.

Using Fortran on this machine, the first thing I wrote was a system to store medical reference information. In the ICU, we had a lot of snippets of tips and tables, like how much blood a patient is allowed to lose the first hours after a coronary bypass, how long to leave a choledochus drain in place, how to calculate cardiac output using the Fick method, and so on[3]. I'd already programmed a Texas Instruments TI-59, one of the earliest programmable calculators, to calcu-

---

[2] Theoretically, this boot loader code should never be overwritten, since there was a hardware lock on that region, but it still happened, and I never figured out why.

[3] I'm not going to explain every medical term here, since it wouldn't add to the story. If you want to know, there's always duckduckgo.com.

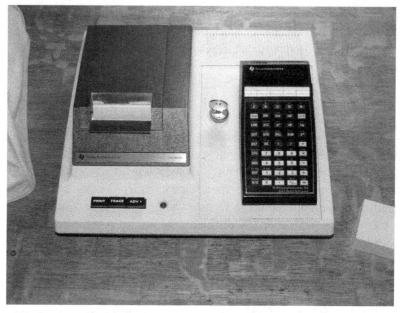

Figure B-2. A TI-59 calculator docked to its PC-100A printer. (Photo Wikimedia Commons, John Crane.)

late cardiac output, pulmonary shunts, and a few more handy things. The TI-59 used little magnetic cards that were fed to the calculator and pulled through it by a motor when you switched programs. For a while, I and the other residents in the ICU used my TI-59, and we passed it from person to person. One of the teaching staff had a PC-100A printer dock, which I used to program some statistics to help with publication work.

With the HP 2100A, I moved those calculations over to the mini computer, added a lot more of our notes of collected wisdom, and set up a terminal in the ICU nursing station. To retrieve information, I figured out an indexing system so that every page of information contained a menu at the bottom leading to other pages. I also built a subscription system so that the residents who "subscribed" to my pages could get a printout of everything that had changed since the last printout they'd gotten.

After this, I wrote a system that used the A/D converter to connect to a bidirectional ultrasound vascular Doppler machine, calculating and graphing a blood flow curve of the aorta. Together with a measurement of the diameter of the aorta, this system could calculate cardiac output without any invasive procedure. Neat and almost accurate enough for clinical use, but not quite.

I also built a tool to make researching medical records somewhat easier. This is the time before we started to disparage retrospective studies, so we still did a lot of those. We researched patient histories to find relationships. Doing this was a lot of work, so I came up with a system that let you set up a list of questions to work through for every medical record studied. Then the answers were fed into the system and you could go play interactively with the data to see what correlated to what. The statistics I implemented were based on the Student's t-test and the chi-square test, and that was pretty much enough. The user selected two different questions from the list of questions, or data points, if you will, then the machine calculated if there was any correlation between the answers for those two questions. It took about ten seconds for a verdict of significance or not to come up on the terminal.

The first study we used this for was a comparison of post-surgery treatments for esophageal cancers. We had quite different results from another university, and we couldn't figure out why. I demonstrated this to Thiery Anné, the lead author of the study [18] one night we were both on call. I grabbed out of thin air what I thought was a ridiculous correlation, comparing the outcome of surgery followed by 5-FU, a chemotherapy agent which we used a lot, depending on location of the cancer (top, middle, or lower esophagus), which I was sure had nothing to do with it. The computer spit out "$p < 0.005$", and Thiery just laughed, saying "yeah, sure, as if THAT would be right... great programming, man!", and wished me luck finding the bug. I spent the next two nights trying to locate the coding error, then finally pulled out all the data, around a hundred patients, and recalculated the whole thing by hand. It all came out exactly the same as the computer had shown. That was the most important finding we had, and it was correct. It explained the difference we saw between the results in our hospital and that other hospital I mentioned, since our patients differed quite clearly in how high in the esophagus the cancer was located. It was also the last time we found anything as spectacular using that system.

During that period I also enrolled for engineering studies, and I got almost two years into it before I had to give it up. There was simply not enough hours in a day, or a night, to do all this.

We did a lot of heart surgeries, sometimes up to three or four in a day, and the main bottleneck was the ICU. Back then, a typical patient stayed on assisted ventilation for up to 24 hours, then had to stay in the ICU another two days or so. We only had a total of six ICU beds for vascular and cardiac patients, so something had to be done about this. Extending the ICU and hiring more nurses was out of the question. Other solutions needed to be found.

Dr. John Kirklin at the University of Alabama had succeeded in reducing the mean length of stay in his ICU down to eight hours by using computers to run the infusion pumps. It turned out that if you continuously adjusted the flow of blood pressure stimulators and blood transfusions automatically according to measured parameters and programmed algorithms, the patient became hemodynamically stable much sooner, and could be taken off the ventilator and moved to medium care much earlier. This is what we wanted to do as well.

I was sent to the USA with two engineers to be trained in the programming of a later operating system version, RTE-IV on the HP 1000 system, a successor to the HP 2100A system I was used to. After that two week course I went on with my wife, but without the engineers, to Birmingham, Alabama, to watch how they did cardiac surgery there.

The idea was that the University of Ghent would also invest in more recent computers, infusion pumps, monitoring, and staff, and do what they'd done in Alabama, increasing the throughput of patients through the ICU, while at the same time reducing complications[4]. But as we got back from the trip we were told that there was no money to spend on equipment or staff. I had figured on a career as a surgeon doing some space-age stuff with computers in the ICU, but it wasn't to be.

In 1983 I quit the university and took over a general practice, patients, house and all. At the same time, I started my first company which initially sold TRS-80 computer games on tapes through mail order. Soon after starting the company, I wrote a very rudimentary home-nursing application on a TRS-80. Then I got an order to write a system to estimate cooling systems for offices and computer rooms, which I did on the EACA Genie-III system. That system ran both NewDOS and CP/M.

---

[4] Anything that reduces time under anesthesia, or time spent in the ICU, is known to reduce infections and other complications.

In the first few years, I sold a number of machines, including the Genie-III machines, Goldstar computers (which were later renamed to LG) and one of the first generation networks (based on TeleVideo mmmOST). I also wrote an accounting program, a program to store patient-record diagnostic codes, and an insurance-agent management program. Mostly, writing these programs served to sell turnkey systems, which was a pretty good business back then. I also programmed and installed a few industrial-control computers from Merlin Systems in the UK. Not much of peripheral electronics was available at that time, so I also designed and built some minor electronics like Whetstone bridges with differential amplifiers for Pt-100 sensors, input-protection circuits, and relay boards.

Around 1987 I arranged a connection to Medline[5] through some organization I've forgotten the name of in Köln in Germany, utilizing packet switching to get there, and a search language I think was called "Diane". When they had a particularly difficult case at the university ICU where I had done my residency, they called me and I did a literature search using my Medline connection, then reported back over fax with a summary of what I found. The very expensive fax machine I sold them for this purpose must have been one of the first fax machines used in that hospital.

I could do a search like this in about an hour's time total. I loved doing this, but it ended a year or two later when the ICU got their own set of Silverplatter's Medline CDROMs to search through. I still think my results were a lot more useful than what they could find on their own, though.

In 1990 I joined "Fidonet" and later ran what was then one of the larger regional nodes[6], using three regular phone lines and an ISDN basic rate connection. Pretty bleeding edge at the time. With the computers I used for this, I also wrote and ran a communication system to deliver lab reports and referral results to general practitioners and specialists. The system was based on the "Fossil 5" communication drivers and used a system I built in the Clarion language

---

[5] Medline is the world's largest collection of medical publications, usually with an abstract, seldom with full text articles. It was the online incarnation of "Index Medicus", the paper-based index of published articles. Medline is part of the US National Library of Medicine.

[6] For the old-timers out there: my node address was 2:291/1906. Now, *that's* some addressing for real men, you DNS huggers!

and assembler to receive files from the labs and deliver them to users when they called in. I actually had a form of end-to-end encryption using symmetric keys that were exclusively stored in a database at each end-user's system. The client application, also written in Clarion, even contained a rudimentary medical records system with daily notes. I only charged the senders for the "stamp"; receivers got the whole thing for free.

This system was pretty darn good for that time, but I had absolutely no patience or talent for marketing, so I never got beyond about ten or 15 subscribers. In 1994 I was approached by a company called "MediBridge" who had the backing of the Belgian telecoms giant Belgacom and the University of Ghent. They had a similar product but built on Solaris systems and packet switching. The end result was way more expensive than my system with less functionality and less reliability. My system's existence had hindered them in several sales where there was always at least one doctor who had seen my system and didn't want theirs. So MediBridge offered me a job and some cash if I let my system die and started working for them instead. This was my way out of my general practice, so I took it with both hands.

During the next year, I was also hired by the University of Ghent to create the Belgian version of the "Episode of Care Summary" specification for electronic messaging interchange. My boss, George De Moor, was then head of the Technical Committee 251 at CEN, the European Standards institution, which led to me being an observer there for almost a year.

During the same period, I became an advisor to the ACC, an organization of around 50 private hospitals in Belgium, to help with the development of their new medical records system, the AZIS-2000. Here I learned from the inside what it is like building a medical record system in an organization that basically had no idea what they were doing, and really couldn't care less. I walked out of there alienated, angry, disappointed, and very disillusioned with vendors of EHR systems.

After a few months of writing a boring and not very good system for care facilities for the elderly, I got a job managing the IT for the department of epidemiology at the Ministry of Health in Brussels. My task there was to migrate them from Windows for Workgroups to NT, while also making them aware of a newfangled thing called "network security", and things like "firewalls". A major reason for hiring me instead of any old IT manager was that the IT people could get absolutely no respect from the doctors that made up most of the users there. The place was like a cat fight, with hissy fits all around, walls of silence alternating with screaming in the hallways, and absolutely nothing being achieved when it came to computing. It was assumed that my medical background would make the users show some respect, and it worked. We did get some order in the house, better equipment, and more security. I loved that job, conflicts and all. The pay was shit, though, it being the government.

I stayed there a year, then went on to "Real Software"[7], where I ended up in a warehouse at Zaventem airport trying to straighten out some really shitty VBA code for half a year. This is where I learned SQL Server pretty well. The next six months after that, I spent writing another medical communications package in C++ with some real asymmetric crypto for use in reporting in a clinical study of some new psychiatric pharmaceutical.

From Real Software, I went to C3, a small startup doing ICU software, where I wrote some of the server-side code in C++ for messaging and for script execution. This lasted until the summer of 2001, when I decided to move back to Sweden.

I got a job at Profdoc AB, one of the major vendors of medical records software in Sweden. My task was to design and implement a communication system allowing transfer of referrals, reports, lab results, and electronic prescriptions between any number of large and small client systems. If you're keeping count, this was the third such system I developed. This one was also based on asymmetric crypto. While my first system was based on Clarion and assembler, and my second system on C++, this system was entirely written in Borland's Delphi, since that was the house language. It took me a little more than three years to build this system, and, as far as I know, it's working just fine still.

In the years that followed, I went back to work as a GP part time in Sweden, while also developing a few minor applications. In 2008 I got hired as a contractor to develop a model application in C# for another division of Profdoc. The idea was to set up an architecture that they could follow when rebuilding some of the legacy applications they had in house. I did this for about one and a half year.

---

[7] How's that for a company name?

In April 2010, I suddenly got the idea of how a medical record should really work, an idea so different from how the EHR systems of today are designed that I simply had to develop a prototype just to see if it could be done. I made the first version of this system which I call "iotaMed" ("Issue Oriented Tiered Architecture for Medicine"), for the iPad in Objective-C. Ever since then I've been refining the idea and writing about it in different media.

I thought the advantages of our iotaMed would be obvious to everyone, but I was wrong. Doctors, in general, understand the idea and find it obviously better and entirely a new thing. They also understand that it is very different from what we have with current EHR systems. Everyone else, that is administrators and developers, seem to understand neither the difference, nor the point. I keep getting the remark that "we already have that", or "nobody ever asked for that", sometimes both at the same time from the same person. This attitude is both infuriating and enlightening. It clearly explains why the systems we keep getting from these administrators and developers are so useless to us. It's as if our (the doctors') way of thinking and working is so alien as to be invisible to them.

I then did what developers always do when met with a seemingly unsolvable problem; I introduced another level of indirection, or as other people say, took a step back. I realized I first needed to explain what the problems were before I could offer the solution. You can't answer a question that hasn't yet been asked.

So this brings us to today and this book. It is intended to provide the right questions for a change, and maybe a few of the answers. I only occasionally touched on the iotaMed design in the book, since that isn't what this book is primarily about. Rest assured, however, iotaMed did result from the thinking that also formed the basis for the book. It's all one and the same thing.

Bibliography

[1] Lawrence L Weed. *Medical records, medical education, and patient care: The problem-oriented record as a basic tool.* Press of Case Western Reserve University, 1970.

[2] Lawrence L Weed and Lincoln Weed. *Medicine in denial.* CreateSpace, 2011.

[3] Garrett P, Seidman J. *EMR vs EHR - What is the Difference?* Health IT Buzz blog, January 4, 2011. http://www.healthit. gov/buzz-blog/electronic-health-and-medical-records/emr-vs-ehr-difference/

[4] Global Polio Eradication Initiative. *Economic Case for Eradicating Polio*, 2013. http://www.polioeradication.org/ Portals/0/Document/Resources/StrategyWork/Economic-Case.pdf

[5] Christopher JL Murray and Julio Frenk. Ranking 37th— measuring the performance of the US healthcare system. *New England Journal of Medicine*, 362(2):98–99, 2010.

[6] American Academy of Family Physicians, AAFP, home page. http://aafp.org

[7] Swedish Institute for Health Services Development (Spri). *Set of Recommendations on Functional Requirements for Healthcare Documentation (1996).* http://www.virtual.epm. br/material/healthcare/A_Reference4.pdf

[8] The Free Dictionary, Medical dictionary. *Problem-Oriented Medical Record (POMR).* Elsevier 2009. http:// medical-dictionary.thefreedictionary.com/Problem-Oriented+Medical+record

[9] Dahlin B. *Från provinsialläkare till primärvård - en historisk exposé.* 2013. http://www.bengtdahlin.se

[10] Hafner K. *A Busy Doctor's Right Hand, Ever Ready to Type.* The New York Times, January 14, 2014. http://www.nytimes. com/2014/01/14/health/a-busy-doctors-right-hand-ever-ready-to-type.html

[11] NIH, U.S. National Library of Medicine. *Fact Sheet MED-LINE.* 2013. http://www.nlm.nih.gov/pubs/factsheets/med-line.html

[12] Bunch C, Dwight J. *Chronic Heart Failure guideline.* http://static.oxfordradcliffe.net/med/gems/CHF.pdf

[13] Wellcome Trust. *Medical Research: What's it worth?* November 2008. http://www.wellcome.ac.uk/stellent/groups/corporatesite/@sitestudioobjects/documents/web_document/wtx052110.pdf

[14] WHO Collaborating Centre for Drug Statistics Methodology. *Anatomical Therapeutic Chemical (ATC) Structure and Principles.* http://www.whocc.no/atc/structure_and_principles/

[15] Atul Gawande. *The checklist manifesto: how to get things right.* Metropolitan Books New York, 2010.

[16] Frederick P Brooks Jr. *The Mythical Man-Month, Anniversary Edition: Essays on Software Engineering.* Pearson Education, 1995.

[17] Teuvo Kohonen. Self-organized formation of topologically correct feature maps. *Biological cybernetics,* 43(1):59–69, 1982.

[18] T Anné, L Berwouts, M Wehlou, G Berzsenyi, and F Derom. Surgical treatment of oesophageal carcinoma. Experience between 1965 and 1980 (author's transl.). *Acta chirurgica Belgica,* 82(4):359, 1982.

Index

A

B

C

finding-issue coefficients 144
fist fights, drunken 28
flowchart representation 62
forms 106
free-form text 99

G

gastroenterologist 29
general template 146
graphing of values 91
guideline 8, 112, 126, 135, 165

H

healthcare issue 92, 127, 153
history field 87
history log 99

I

ICD-10 110
implementation 27
indiscriminate criteria effect 122
information model 69
inheritance 134
initial database 147
initial finding 142, 167
initial inputs 117, 135
interaction 96
interface 27
iotaMed 132, 138
issue 7, 92, 97, 109, 112, 115, 118, 144, 156, 176
issue coefficients 148
issue item 8, 136, 144, 147
issue-oriented medical record 125, 166
issue template 8, 82, 98, 102, 104, 106, 112, 132, 135, 141, 144, 148, 166
issue template block 131
item 8, 127, 136

K

keyhole effect 62, 121
keyword 50, 51, 90, 94, 126, 166
knowledge support 35, 47

www.ingramcontent.com/pod-product-compliance
Lightning Source LLC
LaVergne TN
LVHW050149060326
832904LV00003B/86